This one's for the children of the running and fitness revolutions who stuck their heads through the outer shell and managed to return to a place within sight of the center, especially

> Bill (''Mr. Blood Run''),
> Larry (shooting stars at 400 meters),
> Phil (bagpipes on Cow Mountain), and
> Doug (the Missionary of Emigrant Pass).

CONTENTS

ACKNOWLEDGMENTS

Any nonfiction book results from the assimilation and organization of myriad resources. In the process of gathering such information, especially on a subject as bereft of ready research conclusions as aerobic exercise addiction, the significant bodies of information stand out rather starkly and are much appreciated. The author wishes to thank William Glasser, MD, for his correspondence on the subject of positive—and negative—addiction, and Connie Chan, PhD, for her willingness to share research information on withdrawal from exercise well in advance of its publication in the academic press. The author also wishes to acknowledge Dr. Kenneth Cooper's work in setting straight the record on the death of Jim Fixx. Athletes who were especially helpful in contributing their time and insights include Doug Latimer, Joe Oakes, Paul Asmuth, Dick Collins, and Nancy Ditz. Special thanks to Phil Frank of the *San Francisco Chronicle* for use of his "Farley" cartoon; who is that exercise addict, anyway? The author also wishes to thank Brian Holding of Leisure Press for taking the chance on what, in 1987, appeared to be such an esoteric subject, and editor Peggy Rupert for her editing skills, and for the additional insights gleaned from her trove of personal experiences.

FOREWORD

The Exercise Fix is a remarkable story about how a compulsive need for the next workout can come before family, friends, and work. It is a story about how exercise—a commonly perceived health elixir—can be abused.

And who best to tell the story than a former addict, who was also the leading analyst of the running movement as editor of *Runner's World*. Who best to reveal the keys to recovery than a "reformed runner." Author Richard Benyo takes us on a fascinating journey as he describes how positive addiction to aerobic exercise can turn to negative addiction—and, thank goodness, back to positive addiction.

In the mid-to-late 1970s, runners and other aerobic athletes began reporting trancelike, euphoric feelings of power and happiness arising from their aerobic exercise. Most sport scientists, including me, scoffed at such reports, ascribing them to the lunatic fringe. But the accounts kept accumulating and their credibility grew as the number of aerobic athletes swelled. Was there indeed something to this "runner's (or aerobic) high"?

At the same time that reports of aerobic highs were prevalent among runners, cyclists, swimmers, skiers, and other aerobic athletes, descriptions of these same euphoric feelings began to come from participants and athletes in other sports, in recreational activities, in the performing arts, and in demanding work. These states of mind were labeled experiences or states of "flow."

In the late 1970s, before becoming a publisher, I was a sport psychologist intrigued with what causes people to perform at peak levels. A student of mine, Mary Ann Carmack, introduced me to the reports on runner's high, and we saw the commonality between these reports and those describing the flow experience. We decided to study the aerobic high and addiction to exercise, and what we found was certainly nothing to scoff at—this was a very real and significant phenomenon.

Today much more is known about the causes of the "exercise fix," and Richard Benyo explains them with keen insight—as only one with such intimate personal and professional involvement could. Benyo helps us understand how exercise becomes addictive through the interaction of powerful physical, psychological, and social rewards. I believe that two of those rewards are most significant—the positive consequences of exercise on self-esteem and the mood-altering effects of endorphins, opiates produced by the brain during extended aerobic exercise.

After his fascinating explanation of the ways that exercise can become addictive, Benyo offers help to the millions of exercise addicts. With warmth and sensitivity, this man who loves his exercise fix tells you how to *prevent* negative addiction. And for those who are compulsive exercisers beating their bodies to pieces for a daily dose of endorphins, Benyo offers a sound prescription for beating the aerobic addiction.

Rainer Martens

PREFACE

This book deals with addiction. Not the addiction to crack and cocaine or to prescription drugs that makes the covers of *Time* and *Newsweek*, but still an addiction that can have significant negative effects on a person's life.

Like other addictions, this one is shared by thousands upon thousands of people. Unlike other destructive addictions, there are no treatment centers devoted to it and there is, in fact, little discussion of it. When mentioned at all, it is mentioned in phrases steeped in positive connotations. It is more bragged about than whispered about.

Adding to its allure is the fact that, unlike cocaine and alcohol and prescription drugs, it costs little in real dollars. But this addiction, like others, becomes the addict's life focus, an all-consuming passion.

It is the addiction to exercise.

It sounds overly dramatic to speak of addiction to aerobic exercise in the same breath with potentially debilitating addictions to drugs, but those who've experienced aerobic addiction know that it can lead to starkly similar dead ends.

Aerobic addiction on a remarkable scale is a relatively new phenomenon linked directly to the increase in the pursuit of aerobic sports such as running, bicycling, long-distance swimming, cross-country skiing, and aerobic dance as a means to better health. It is a phenomenon wherein a person's next aerobic workout becomes the central focus in life.

This book is the end result not only of watching amateur aerobic athletes become slavishly addicted to their workouts, but of being one of them. It also reflects the findings of various scientists on the subject of aerobic addiction.

It examines the process by which aerobic athletes become "hooked" on their sport to the point that it becomes a negative influence in their lives by usurping the positions of family, friends, job, and even personal health. It presents self-tests to help the reader determine if commitment to an aerobic sport has progressed to compulsion. It also suggests a method of avoiding what I've come to call the *physicality syndrome*, while also outlining ways to escape that condition without giving up the benefits of participation in aerobic sports.

In 1976 I weighed 207 pounds. To kids who had grown up with me and hadn't seen me in a decade, the fact that I had gained so much weight was astonishing. In my senior year in high school (1963-64) I'd had trouble topping 150 pounds on my 6-foot frame.

The weight gain was due to several factors, the foremost of which was that I'd ended up with office jobs (first as a newspaper editor, then as a magazine editor) that demanded 70 and more hours a week of work and that allowed little time for exercise. In high school I'd been very active physically; in the workaday world, I was active mentally but physically stalled.

In 1976 a former high school classmate died. He was a heavy smoker, heavy drinker, heavy eater, and was heavily into depression. His death at age 31 shocked me into taking a good look at my own lack of physical condition.

I'd run cross-country in college and decided that I would rekindle my interest in running as a means of getting into shape. I could not psychologically face running until I was below 200 pounds, however. On my birthday in April of 1977 I went on a diet—a very simple diet. I cut out lunch and ate an apple instead. In less than 2 months I was down to 199. The day was June 13, 1977.

I huffed and puffed twice around the block. I sat around for a half hour gasping. When sufficiently recovered, I took a shower—a long shower. I did the same thing the next day, and the next. Gradually, I increased my distance. Within 6 weeks I had done a long run of 5 miles.

During this period I learned of a job opening as managing editor at a magazine in California called *Runner's World*. I applied. And got the job.

I started on August 1. Inspired by covering a marathon from the press truck in October, I decided to train for and run a marathon. Six months later, in April of 1978, I ran my first marathon. In May of 1978 I ran my second marathon. In June I did my third marathon. By the end of 1978 I had run eight marathons and had done a few ultramarathons for good measure.

Sometimes I didn't get my daily run in until 11 o'clock at night, and then it might be in the middle of a rainstorm. (Incredibly, I found that I was *not* the only one out running under those conditions.) But I always got the workout in. As a result of the workouts, it was almost always difficult to step out of bed onto the floor in the morning because of sore and stiff Achilles tendons. Compared to the tendons, the blisters and black toenails and shinsplints were nothing.

But I kept running. I *needed* to run. And I had plenty of company with whom I could run and race. The period from 1977 through 1980 saw an explosion of long-distance runners. Most of them were, like myself, members of the "baby boomer" generation, seemingly on a maniacal quest to arrest youth. The running had gone beyond arresting youth, however. It had become a sort of therapy, a way to deal with the uncertainties of life, an escape, a window in the day through which we could crawl into a more pleasant world.

After the first awkward, stilted, painful mile of the day, the muscles would warm up, the body rhythm would kick in, the mind would unhinge, and the worries of daily life would slip away.

It became apparent that running had become a sort of psychological fix we hungrily anticipated and needed each day. We talked passionately of our love of running and of our commitment to it: how we would certainly do this for the rest of our lives. We ran more and more, we ran through aches and pains and eventually through injuries. We saw ourselves as enlightened, a sweatsuited society of special souls who had found "The Answer."

Eventually, however, the injuries we'd tried to ignore began to overtake us, and we were hobbled. And once hobbled, we suffered withdrawal symptoms. Podiatrists dealing with injured runners began to routinely apply casts to the runners' legs because if they didn't, the runners would run anyway, drawn compulsively to get in their daily fix.

From my position at *Runner's World* I was able to observe that this phenomenon was not peculiar to our little running group. It was surprisingly common among runners all over the country. And, by extending my gaze a bit more, I found it was not uncommon in other aerobic sports, especially in bicycling, in the then-emerging sport of the triathlon, and in the wildly growing world of aerobic dance.

I accidentally slipped off the compulsion train in 1980 by setting a goal of running a sub-3-hour marathon. The quest involved radically changing my training by adding regular doses of speed workouts at the track and by limiting my long, slow distance workouts to two or three times a week. From this new perspective of a carefully followed program that included rest days, what I *had* been doing with my running began to appear unhealthy.

I began observing the dark side of the compulsive, addicted runner. I had enough research to start with: My friends and I had been more than compulsive and addictive ourselves. I quickly found, however, that there were increasing numbers of clinical studies on aerobic commitment, aerobic addictions, endorphin release, and the like.

What follows is the integration of published research on the subject and my own experiences and observations of what I've come to regard as *The Exercise Fix*.

—Richard Benyo
St. Helena, California

1
CHAPTER

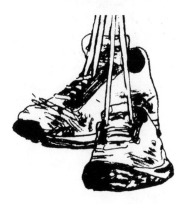

DEFINING
THE EXERCISE FIX

A regular program of aerobic endurance exercise is very beneficial to the cardiovascular system; the system that includes the heart, the lungs, and the circulation. "It is this type of long, steady endurance exercise which is associated with benefits to the cardiovascular system," wrote Terence Kavanagh, MD (1986, p. 66), pioneer in the use of jogging to rehabilitate heart patients.

Regular aerobic exercise as practiced by millions of Americans has been instrumental over the past decade in stalling, and in fact reversing, the statistical incidence in the United States of death due to heart disease. One study piles upon the next in glorifying regular aerobic exercise and good nutrition as the best way to increase general health and to fight heart disease.

The term *aerobics* became common language in 1968 with the publication of *Aerobics*, by Kenneth Cooper, MD, which presented a simple-to-follow program of endurance exercise based upon a weekly point system. The program was predicated upon the best evidence of the time that the development of heart disease, the number one killer of adult Americans, could be influenced by a modest program of mild but continuous exercise. Jogging, which Cooper cited with running as the simplest form of aerobic exercise, became the backbone of his program.

Thousands of middle-aged Americans, particularly business executives, took up Cooper's program and achieved lower risks of heart disease, effective weight control, and physical self-esteem.

In the wake of Frank Shorter's victory in the Olympic marathon in 1972, Shorter's contemporaries (the "baby boomers," a generation younger than Cooper's followers) began in ever-greater numbers to take up long-distance running in an attempt to look and feel younger. This "running revolution" peaked between 1976 and 1980.

The revolution expanded into the fitness revolution in 1980 and hasn't slowed since. The 1987 Gallup Leisure Activities Index indicates that 12 percent of adult Americans jog, 26 percent of those every day. A notable number of Americans have enthusiastically taken up aerobic dancing, bicycling, and cross-country skiing. The triathlon, an event combining running, swimming, and biking, was invented in the 1970s and is experiencing continually growing participation. The Gallup poll found that in 1987 some 49 percent of all Americans claimed to follow *some* fitness regimen, up from 20 percent in 1961.

As the number of Americans taking part in aerobic and endurance sports increased in the 1970s, William Glasser, MD, founder of the Institute for Reality Therapy in Los Angeles, observed a phenomenon that he termed *positive addiction* (1976). He studied long-distance runners and found that they faithfully pursued what would seem to the uninitiated a rather boring occupation, but that they were able to persist because they became "addicted" to it. Glasser referred to this addiction as positive to differentiate it from the classic negative addictions to alcohol and drugs. Addiction to long-distance running could be viewed as positive because the addiction did so many good things for the runner's body and psyche. In fact, the positive addiction to running—and, by inference, to any aerobic sport—was so beneficial that it was even responsible for some people being able to kick a negative addiction by taking up running as a sort of substitute.

An excellent example of this is found in Tim Joe Key, a San Diego runner and founder of the hard-core ultrarunning club, The Flatlanders. Before he discovered distance running and used it as a centering point, Key led a life on the downslide. He was incarcerated a number of times, once for a murder he didn't commit, and he had a three-pack-a-day cigarette habit. In 1970, after an Army hitch, he went to college, graduating in 1977 at age 33. That year, after an incident in which he began coughing up brown phlegm, he quit smoking and took up running. In 1978 he completed the Mission Bay Marathon in 3-1/2 hours. His weight had dropped from 215 to 165. "Running is my emotional safety valve," he said.

Subsequent research into just what happens within the human body that could make such a seemingly boring pursuit as running so palatable to otherwise intelligent people uncovered natural opiate-like substances—endorphins—that are produced by the brain to mask pain and discomfort. Many amateur runners had recounted instances during some runs of a blissful, almost trancelike state that came to be known as "the runner's high," which was later linked to the release of the brain's pain-dulling drugs.

With hundreds of thousands of Americans running around in little more than their underwear pursuing healthy hearts, slimmer bodies, and increased self-esteem, scientists had enough subjects from whom to draw information on the real and imagined effects of sustained aerobic activity.

Among the growing ranks of runners, however, were some exhibiting negative symptoms. Foremost among those symptoms were what medical professionals call *overuse injuries*. These are injuries, usually to the lower extremities, caused by chronic use—and misuse—of the same muscles, tendons, cartilage, and ligaments. Because few of the hundreds of thousands of runners taking up the sport had coaches to rein them in and to set them on rational training programs, many overdid their exercise and ended up injured. Typically, the white-collar professionals who fueled the running boom were used to pushing the pace in life and frequently transferred this tendency to a sport that requires gradual buildups of training loads on unused muscle systems.

Another negative symptom that I observed from my position as executive editor of *Runner's World* was a tendency for new runners to become preoccupied with running to the point that they would run despite nagging injuries, would run compulsively, would become obsessed with mileage and with the regularity of their training runs, and would talk and think about running to the exclusion of almost all else.

I groped with what to call the phenomenon and originally called it *physicality*, which is a tendency to stress the physical above all else, and often to the exclusion of all else. The word physicality did not exactly roll off the tongue, however, and eventually I found myself referring more frequently to Glasser's book *Positive Addiction* (1976).

That, combined with the increasingly sophisticated research to isolate the pain-dulling endorphin and to describe its effects upon the exercising individual, nudged my thinking toward identifying a class beyond Glasser's positive addiction group that I considered calling the *positive negative addicts.* In my mind, the phrase referred to people who'd become involved in running and other aerobic sports as a positive addiction and then had allowed the sport, for whatever reason, to become such an obsession that it had turned into a negative factor in their lives.

Finally, however, the phrase *exercise fix* began to emerge as the most easily understood term. It made no immediate value judgment of a person's involvement, while still making the point that some sort of an addiction was involved. When I tried the term out on exercisers and nonexercisers, they were more likely to know what I meant: that compulsion among regular aerobic exercisers to get out there to receive their daily dose of exercise, no matter what.

For this book, the exercise fix refers to an aerobic athlete's compulsive need for the next workout, not necessarily to improve performance in competition but to provide relief from the bad feelings associated with *not* working out.

FARLEY/Phil Frank

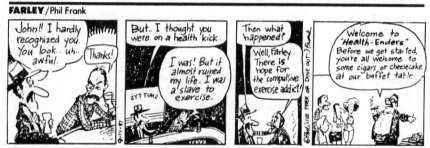

Reprinted by permission of Phil Frank/*San Francisco Chronicle.*

COMMITMENT OR COMPULSION?

In order to develop and maintain aerobic (cardiovascular) fitness, a person must practice the aerobic activity on a regular basis. Kenneth Cooper, father of aerobics, considers doing a 20-minute workout three or four times a week, or every other day, to be practicing aerobic fitness on a regular basis.

Aerobic practitioners who go beyond Cooper's minimum recommendations tend to participate in the activity for reasons other than good cardiovascular health. They find fulfillment in the fitness activity itself and not merely in the end result, which becomes a sort of by-product.

These more ambitious people tend to invest a good deal of time and commitment in training and racing, whether the aerobic activity is long-distance running or swimming, sustained bicycling, cross-country skiing, aerobic dance, or the triathlon. Generally, these are laudable pursuits that provide an extreme degree of fitness to the athlete and provide an arena for socially acceptable personal fulfillment.

A number of these people, however, consistently escalate their fitness pursuits until those pursuits become the center of their lives, displacing family, friends, sex, hobbies, and job in importance. The admonition that "too much of anything is not good for you" comes forcibly into play.

The following self-test is designed to gauge your attitude toward your involvement in aerobic pursuits. Some of the questions may not be applicable to you at this time in your aerobic career. For instance, you may never have consulted a sports therapist or sports psychologist, and to you the statement, "My sports therapist is my best friend," may seem rather absurd. Consequently, you will likely place a score of 1 next to it.

Some of the statements refer to a specific type of aerobic pursuit (the triathlon) but are applicable to a variety of aerobic efforts, and presumably you will answer accordingly. Other statements are general: "If you don't even try, you've already lost." These have an obvious application to aerobic activities, and especially to aerobic competition.

A Self-Test
Where Exercise Addiction Stands in Your Life

On a scale of 1 to 10, with 10 being the strongest, give an objective weight to each of the following statements as they apply to you and your endurance fitness. Then total your numbers and see the interpretations at the end of the test. Fill the test out with pencil, or make photocopies so you can retake it periodically.

_____ Aerobic fitness is important to me. I'm positive I'll be engaged in one or more endurance sports for the rest of my life.

_____ A day without an endurance workout is like a day without sunshine.

_____ If it becomes downright impossible to get my workout in today, I can always double up tomorrow.

_____ Until I get my workout in, I'm a real "bear"—as in "unbearable."

_____ A little pain proves there's progress being made.

_____ If 5 hours of workout a week is good, 10 hours is twice as good.   (Cont.)

Continued

_____ Warm-up and cool-down are important, but it's what comes in the middle of a workout that counts.

_____ As far as endurance training goes, more is always better.

_____ "My workouts for the past week? Glad you asked—!"

_____ Regularity at any cost is the backbone of all fitness.

_____ Quality without quantity is wasteful.

_____ "My sports therapist is my best friend."

_____ You're not a real runner until you've done a marathon.

_____ Triathlons are important because they allow you to do more training with impunity.

_____ To go for more, always for more, is what's important in life.

_____ Rest is for the weary, not for the strong.

_____ An unbroken string of workouts should remain so.

_____ A person who has nothing to prove has already made a point.

_____ If you don't even try, you've already lost.

_____ Relaxation is all right _after_ you've made the grade.

_____ TOTAL YOUR SCORE.

Where does your total fall? 161-200, exercise addiction personified; 121-160, leanings toward exercise addiction; 81-120, nearly neutral; 41-80, fitness with a mellow bent; 10-40, approaching terminal mellow. Retake this test every 4 to 6 months.

Analyzing Your Score

What was your total for the test?

Let's briefly examine the various levels of involvement in aerobic activities indicated by the test results:

20-40. Very few people involved in aerobic activities are likely to score this low simply because, to pursue an aerobic activity, a certain commitment to regularity is necessary. Consequently, answering the first question truthfully is likely to put the typical aerobic exerciser well on the way to the next level.

41-80. A person who pursues aerobic fitness according to Cooper's minimum weekly requirements and who maintains fitness strictly for its health benefits is likely to fall into this category.

81-120. This range is referred to as neutral because it includes people who occasionally increase their training to take part in an annual competition or two or who typically increase their involvement in aerobic activities when the weather improves. People in this category tend to stay involved in aerobic fitness all year round, but to escalate the involvement on occasion as the spirit or season moves them.

121-160. Most aerobic athletes fall into this category. They are involved in fitness for more than just the health benefits, and they regularly pursue competitive goals, whether that means trying to break 40 minutes in the 10K road race or doing three or four short-course triathlons per summer. This group also includes aerobic dancers who periodically gear up to reach higher levels and bicyclists who regularly train for and take part in century rides and other endurance events. Also included are cross-country skiers who compete in several citizens' races a year.

161-200. At this level one's commitment to aerobic activities and sports tends to cross over into obsessive and compulsive behavior. Aerobic training becomes more important than nearly anything else in life. It is the focal point of each day. There is a tendency to willingly train through injuries and to compete in races when injured. There is also a tendency to blindly defend one's intense involvement on the basis of the benefits aerobic fitness bestows on the human body. The phrase ''No pain, no gain'' is used at first to get through difficult workouts, and later to justify training while injured.

It is advisable to retake the self-test periodically because, as with other addictions, aerobic involvement may go through peaks and valleys, binges and layoffs (often occasioned by temporarily debilitating injuries associated with the fitness activity).

The more typical tendency, however, is for the person addicted to aerobic exercise to pursue that exercise in a headstrong and headlong fashion.

Let us examine the relatively recent phenomenon of thousands of people allowing a good love to go bad.

COMMITMENT AMONG DEDICATED AEROBIC ATHLETES

As I mentioned in the preface, during the height of the running revolution there was a great deal of talk about commitment.

We were all so enthusiastically involved in running, had gotten so much from running, both physically and psychologically, that we were convinced we would be blissfully running for the rest of our lives. We were deeply committed to running—we loved it. It was *literally* a love affair: Running had been so good to us that we would never desert it.

Looking back a decade later, it is easy to find our wild enthusiasm at once naive and unrealistic. Naive because our enthusiasm knew no bounds; it was almost like puppy love. In a sense, it *was* puppy love for a part of ourselves we had begun to feel was forever lost. It was unrealistic because the typical human body is unable to hold up under the assault of so many glorious workouts.

In previous generations, once you left high school and moved on, either to the working world or to college (and thence to the working world), your childhood, your adolescence was over. What faced you was a lifetime of work, commitment to raising a family, responsibilities. In essence, childhood's end.

For the baby boomer generation, the prospects were doubly bleak. First, many of that generation were going to college, unlike their parents, and were training for white-collar jobs that were typically salaried (requiring unpaid overtime) and typically sedentary: There were no physical demands, which meant that the 22-year-old body was going to be allowed to rust. The second factor was the incredible media barrage surrounding the concept of a ''youth culture'' that was foisted on the baby boomers by Madison Avenue during the 1960s. The baby boomers had made an impact during that decade and had sparked changes in government policies with their antiwar protests. The youth had stood up and had been counted. But in standing up, they had become an easy target.

Ironically, the goddess Youth as presented by Madison Avenue was turning out to be an unfaithful harlot.

It became incredibly difficult to maintain one's youth while working 50- and 60-hour weeks in entry-level white-collar jobs. This difficulty was further compounded by the inevitability of aging. Warned during the 1960s to trust no one over 30, we were rapidly approaching 30 ourselves.

Enter long-distance running: an avocation that required little in the way of talent or equipment. It required no club membership. It required no scheduling of a partner. It required no elaborate or expensive sports complex—it could be done in the road.

Suddenly, an hour a day of running could stall aging, extend youth, provide exercise and fitness, counter sedentary body fat, increase energy reserves, release tension, provide a soon-to-be socially acceptable way of having fun, offer camaraderie, and so on. It was nirvana. And the more you did it, the easier it seemed to become. No wonder so many baby boomers followed Olympic marathoner Frank Shorter down the winding road paved with the promise of extended youth.

Besides being naively willing to fall deeply in love with this old and wonderful activity and to speak of life-long commitment, we were unrealistic about the very consequences of that commitment, which can be listed simply:

1. *Physical injury.* Such unbridled running on such untried legs would eventually lead to overuse injuries, and that unbridled enthusiasm would typically aggravate the injuries by restarting running before the injury was healed properly, thus leading to additional injuries.

2. *Family commitments.* As a generation, the white-collar baby boomers were late in starting families. They sometimes got married right out of school but tended to put off having children often for many years. This pattern was due to several factors. One was that both husband and wife had professions and therefore jobs, and in an age of growing feminism, there was reluctance for the wife to give up her job to start a family. Also, two incomes provided a standard of living that many young couples were not anxious to trade for the dubious satisfaction of being parents. And there was that desperate holding on to youth: To have a family was to symbolically take that first inexorable step into middle age. But that step *was* inexorable, and the subsequent responsibilities cut into training time.

3. *Enthusiasm maintenance.* The level of enthusiasm most baby boomers brought to their running could not possibly be maintained over the long haul. Even with all the benefits a running lifestyle provided, one's enthusiasm had to be channelled into other pressing areas: job, personal relationships, personal finance, and the like.

The incredible commitment expressed by the runners I knew during the 1978-80 period, and my own commitment, felt genuine; in hindsight, however, the commitment was not very realistic.

It might be argued that my view of the situation was rather narrow. I observed this pattern in a small group of runners with whom I trained and raced.

Actually, the view was anything but narrow. As executive editor of *Runner's World*, I had access to literally hundreds of thousands of runners who were as committed as I was, and sometimes more. *Runner's World* had a very strong subscription base at that time: long-distance runners who had the magazine delivered to their homes every month. The *Runner's World* subscriber was an advertiser's dream. Demographic studies that the magazine commissioned over the years came back with consistently glowing reports: The subscribers were young, professional, upscale, highly educated.

And, because of their education combined with their enthusiasm, *Runner's World* subscribers were prone to writing letters. The volume of mail during those years was overwhelming. And nearly every letter was drenched with commitment to the sport.

The holding company that owned *Runner's World* also published other magazines for aerobic athletes. As I became editorial director of the company, I learned quickly that, although what was happening with running was unique in the history of sport because of the skyrocketing numbers, similar feelings were being expressed by readers of *Bike World* and *Nordic World* (for cross-country skiers). The enthusiasm for and commitment to aerobic sports, especially once the advocate went beyond the dabbling stages and became serious, were overwhelming. As the triathlon emerged as a sport, a similar fanaticism grew in that arena.

Ironically, this almost blind enthusiasm among amateur aerobic practitioners was not shared by professional athletes. *Runner's World* annually sponsored what was known as National Running Week, a full week between Christmas and New Year's Day of seminars, clinics, races, and so on, that brought the enthusiastic new runners together with the heroes and heroines of the sport. A pattern emerging in conversation with many of the professional athletes suggested that when their competitive careers were over, they'd be extremely happy to hang up the racing flats and never run another step. This was not true with *all* professional runners, but it was common among a surprising majority of them, including Derek Clayton, Herb Elliott, and others.

Over the years, it became apparent that although the average enthusiastic, committed amateur runner could line up in the same race with the pros, there was a world of difference between them. The professional distance runner seemed motivated by competition, while the amateur seemed motivated by training. This difference would become increasingly stark as thousands of Americans continued to pour into the ever-growing pool of committed runners.

The larger the number, the more obvious the patterns of commitment became. And consequently, the more obvious became the patterns of over-commitment.

THE TASK OF MEASURING COMMITMENT

Whereas it is easy to measure a person's height and weight, measuring a person's commitment is not a straightforward task. Commitment is very much subjective. An extremely committed 1972 Nixon campaign worker might have had second thoughts about continuing to dedicate massive physical and emotional energy to someone who condoned breaking into the Democratic headquarters at the Watergate Hotel. Similarly, a preteen's vow in 1968 that she was committed body and soul to the bubblegum rock group The Archies might not have rung true by the time she turned 30.

Most of the hundreds of thousands of Americans in their 30s who found long-distance running in 1978 believed from the bottom of their soles that they were fully committed to running as a sport, a lifestyle, and a future. They saw the good things it did for them, and they were prepared to make a heartfelt commitment. They had the best of intentions when they made their enthusiastic declarations, but in many cases, reality eventually stepped in and derailed their commitment.

The growing number of people becoming involved in long-distance running and, subsequently, in other aerobic sports did not go unnoticed by the professionals who note and comment on such things. Long before the running craze was cited in *Time* and *Newsweek*, two medical doctors were sufficiently intrigued by the phenomenon to write books about it.

Glasser saw *Positive Addiction* published in 1976. The book explored the concept that transcendental meditation and jogging offered positive psychological benefits and that both activities, especially jogging, had addictive qualities that made it relatively easy for a person to get hooked while benefiting greatly from the experience. This situation was opposed to negative addictions, which appealed to weaknesses in people and which further catered to those weaknesses, undermining any strength a person might hope to muster to deal with life.

The other major book on running was *The Joy of Running* (1976) by psychiatrist Thaddeus Kostrubala, MD. Unlike the Glasser book, which brought together a fairly complex theory, Kostrubala's book brought together the currently perceived physical benefits of a three-times-a-week running program. Kostrubala explained how to begin and maintain a running program, outlined the physical benefits, and in later chapters touched on the addictive characteristics of the avocation and the psychological benefits of continued long-distance running. An enthusiastic runner himself, Kostrubala used running as a form of therapy with some of his patients. His personal enthusiasm can be seen in the final chapter of the book, which is dedicated to the marathon, and his personal quests in the 26.2-mile distance.

Both Glasser and Kostrubala cited numerous examples of the "altered state of consciousness" that leads to the fabled *runner's high* (see chapters 2 and 3 of this book), and both cited elevated levels of commitment to running by patients they'd treated and runners they'd interviewed and surveyed in questionnaires.

Science is not grown on speculation and theory, however. Two researchers at the University of Illinois at Urbana-Champaign, Mary Ann Carmack and Rainer Martens, enthusiastic runners themselves, set out to study runners and their commitment to the running lifestyle. The result was a 1979 paper titled "Measuring Commitment to Running: A Survey of Runners' Attitudes and Mental States."

The Carmack and Martens research, conducted in southern Illinois, involved 315 runners, 250 males and 65 females. The median age was 28.8. Some 82 percent of the 315 runners fell into one of four groups:

1. Competitive amateur road racers
2. High school track athletes at a track camp
3. University of Illinois personnel who jogged at lunch
4. Potential Olympic middle- and long-distance runners

The study found that the more regularly the runners ran, and the more often they ran longer than 40 minutes, the more committed they were to running, the more addicted they perceived themselves to be, and the more discomfort they felt when they missed a scheduled run.

The results of the study confirmed what Glasser and Kostrubala had observed among their patients and among their running acquaintances. Additionally, both Glasser and Kostrubala had indicated that one had to run 40 minutes or beyond in order to attain the state described as the runner's high. The Carmack and Martens study confirmed that finding with its own more scientific results.

The Carmack and Martens study likewise held no real surprises when it came to reasons for beginning running, reasons for presently running, and outcomes derived from running. The following are the top three answers in each category:

Reasons for beginning running
1. Maintain fitness
2. Enjoyment
3. Lose weight

Reasons for presently running
1. Maintain fitness
2. Enjoyment
3. Competition

Outcomes derived from running
1. Feel better
2. Cardiovascular endurance
3. Provide a challenge

The fact that people who said they were committed to running was validated scientifically caused no great ripples in the aerobic pond. What was interesting in the study, however, were the several indications of extreme commitment, a confirmation of the tendency to become addicted to the sport, and reports of feelings of guilt and depression associated with missing scheduled runs.

WHEN COMMITMENT TURNS TO COMPULSION

According to Robert Hirschfeld, MD, a psychiatrist in charge of the Affective and Anxiety Disorders Research Branch of the National Institute of Mental Health in Rockville, Maryland, about 3.5 million adult Americans are victims of obsessive-compulsive behavior to the extent that they cannot function in daily life. Some 300,000 children also suffer from a socially debilitating form of obsessive-compulsive behavior. "It grossly interferes with people's lives," Hirschfeld said. "They become totally unable to function" (Lunder, 1988, p. E1).

Many more Americans exhibit obsessive-compulsive tendencies but are not so susceptable to the accompanying urges that they are unable to function. According to Eric Hollander of Columbia University's Anxiety Disorders Clinic, quoted in the same article, people with mild obsessive-compulsive disorders can be very successful in life. "A small amount of worry helps you plan ahead; a small amount of compulsiveness helps you strive for perfection," he said (Lunder, p. E2).

There are many theories to explain the origins of obsessive-compulsive behavior. Some of the most prominent theories were cited in the same article by Wayne Goodman, a psychiatrist at Yale University. Those theories are as follows:

1. The problem can begin in childhood. A child pushed to the point of anxiety about everything he or she does by overly strict parents, a rigid educational system (a military academy, for instance), or an unusually strict religious upbringing can develop obsessive-compulsive behavior.

2. The disease has also been associated with birth trauma, such as a temporary lack of oxygen.

3. There is some association with Tourette's syndrome, which indicates that the problem *can* be inherited. Studies indicate that fully half the people with Tourette's also suffer from obsessions and compulsions.

4. Some studies indicate that an altered pattern of blood flow in the brain can cause obsessive-compulsive behavior. There is a connection with the brain chemical serotonin, which at proper levels provides a feeling of certainty, but which at heightened levels or when a person has heightened sensitivity can cause compulsive behavior.

I take the time and space to outline these possible causes of obessive-compulsive behavior because, as we shall see later, a little compulsiveness can lead one to become hooked on an aerobic sport, especially in the presence of positive reinforcement (both physical and mental) and an endorphin release in the brain during workouts.

Obsessive-compulsive behavior is also discussed because one must be able to draw a line where commitment ends and compulsion begins. Drawing that line is at once easy and difficult. It is easy if one is objective and says simply that commitment turns to compulsion when the activity produces negative events, forces, or habits in one's life. The difficulty comes with subjectivity: It is hard to recognize the aerobic activity's negative aspects if one is heavily engaged in the activity and is therefore blinded to those negative aspects.

Some real-life examples can help illuminate the problem. I'd like you to meet four athletes.

Joe Oakes

I first met Joe Oakes shortly after I moved to California in 1977 to work at *Runner's World* magazine. Each Sunday morning *Runner's World* would sponsor Fun-Runs at the local junior college that were noncompetitive runs at various distances. Joe was at every race; in fact, on weekends when the magazine staff had to be out of town on business, Joe would officiate at the races. We'll let Joe tell his story.

"When I was about 40 years old, I weighed over 200 pounds. I began exercising at that point on doctor's orders. But I found that I enjoyed it. The more I did, the more I enjoyed it. I ran quarter miles to start off with, because that's as far as I could go. Then 5 miles, and then 10Ks and marathons. By nature I'm more of a sprinter. But I found I enjoyed myself *more* with the 5-milers than with the sprints, and I'd go out and run them hard. Later I enjoyed running the marathons much the same way. Then the ultramarathons. Each thing that I did gave me a bit of a taste of something more than I'd done before. I guess 'more' is the word. You look at what you've done, and you say, 'Hey, I've done that. What's next? What other accomplishment is there?'

"I became a glutton for exercise. Then I tried what I thought was the ultimate, the Western States 100-Mile Endurance Run, and that was no big deal. The first time out, I got my belt buckle [a silver belt buckle is presented to everyone who finishes in less than 24 hours], so I thought, 'Well, maybe there's something besides running.'

"That's when I started doing triathlons, and because triathlons were just being born in those days, unknowingly, I started at the top. I started with the [Hawaii] Ironman, which was the first triathlon I ever did.

"I've always been the kind of person, in business and in everything, who looks for a way to fit best into what you can do best. I've done that in business and been very successful. And I've done that in athletics and been very successful.

"But I think I overdid it on triathlons. I did the Ironman six times. I got into triathlons because there's a lot more variety associated with it; there's a lot less opportunity for boredom out there, and a lot less opportunity for personal injury. If you *do* injure yourself in running, you've got to stop running, but if you're training for different sports and you injure yourself in running, then you cycle or swim. You're never completely out of it, unless you have a catastrophic accident.

"I *did* have a catastrophic accident, and I was so badly into my training and competing, that 8 days after breaking three ribs, my shoulder, and my wrist [he was struck by a car while training on his bicycle], I went and did the Ironman anyway. I did the swim with my left arm, and the bike and run weren't quite so difficult. There was pain associated with it, but that's what aspirin are for.

"When I came home from that, I thought: 'Oakes, you must be f----n' crazy.' And I guess I realized that I was."

Today Oakes trains more sensibly, although he still claims he stays at a level of fitness where he could run a marathon at the drop of a hat.

Doug Latimer

Latimer was the publisher of *Women's Sports and Fitness*. In 1977-78 he was an executive with *Runner's World*, where he had come from Harper & Row. He had discovered running almost by accident while at Harper & Row and discovered that he was fairly good at it. He became rather obsessed with the Western States 100, an event that is ranked as the most grueling endurance event in the world by *Outside* magazine. As of 1988, Doug had run Western States 12 times, more than any other person. He won it once, and placed in the top eight on 9 of his first 10 attempts; on his one failure to place in the top eight, he had to be carried off the course near the 70-mile point. When he raced in the 1988 edition, he was 50 years of age.

"There probably were times when I would duck out for running at lunch when I should have stayed at my desk and written another memo or another letter or sold another ad. But I would take the Western States 100 so seriously that, by God, if I had to do a double trail run tonight up in the hills because it was part of my training schedule, and if I don't do it I know I can't get it in because it is too close to another difficult run, I would get out of here and I would do it. Even though I'm normally a mild-mannered guy, nothing makes me madder than if I'm really training and something is getting in the way of my training run. It gets me very angry. I get furious! Livid! I have changed my attitude a lot, though.

"I have become more casual, and even though Western States is still my main goal, I'm not as compulsive. I have learned, for example, that not only is it okay to take a day off in the middle of serious training, it's very beneficial to take some time off. Your body recovers much better

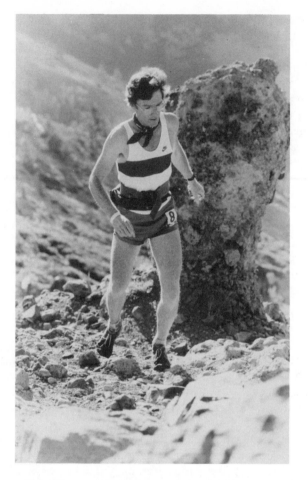

Doug Latimer, "Mr. Western States," negotiates the Sierra Nevada Mountains in one of his 9 outings. (Hughes Photography)

if you don't run at all the day after a hard run. I used to run 3 or 4 months training for Western States at maybe 125 miles a week and never missed a day. If I knew then what I know now, I would probably have won the race 4 years in a row. But because of a combination of stupid training, stupid pacing, and stupid nutrition, I lost at least two of the races. Right now I have pretty good perspective regarding my running. I want to keep running because I love it and because it is healthy. It is an important part of my life's plan. So I value it for that reason; I'm no longer compulsive about it."

Linda Buchanan

Linda Buchanan went to college at the University of California in San Diego. She was very athletic—running, swimming, skiing, playing tennis. In 1980 she began cycling regularly in preparation for her first triathlon. She placed second among the women. By 1983 she was one of the youthful sport's top competitors, with major wins in Nice, France, and Kauai, Hawaii.

At that time she lived in Davis, California. Her training fell into a pattern: 2 to 3 hours cycling, an hour swimming, and an hour running. She had no coach; she consistently redid what had worked for her the previous week.

"It was just work out, work out, work out," she told *Outside* Magazine writer John Brant (1986). "I felt there was nothing new to conquer. I started to lose my desire and motivation. Every time I went out to train I was in considerable pain. But a large part of excelling in this sport is putting up with pain, so I would try to keep going, which only made things worse. It became a cycle. I lost the ability to distinguish between discomfort and pain. I just couldn't register that difference" (Brant, p. 70).

In late spring of 1984 Buchanan went to Santa Barbara to train in the coastal hills. "I'd wake up and could barely walk," she said. "All I could do was just drag my left leg around" (p. 71). When she consulted a doctor at her father's insistence, she learned she had an extremely serious stress fracture in her left leg, where a cavity had opened in the bone and a leg muscle had ruptured its lining.

Buchanan went into a 6-month sports hiatus while the leg healed. "It was horrible," she said. "After all the years of being active, all the tennis and swimming and running, I was completely cut off for the first time. It made me realize how much sports were a part of my life" (p. 112). She returned to become the United States Triathlon Society's champion in 1985 and has managed to compete at a high level without reverting to a compulsive training pattern.

Bruce Dern

Bruce Dern was quite a good half-miler in college. I interviewed him in 1977 for *Runner's World*, and he had a tremendous memory for running facts and figures—and an equally tremendous need to run. He admitted to being obsessive about the sport. His daily mileage would vary between 5 and 10 miles, and some days he still worked out on the track with an intensity that hadn't dimmed since high school. He also occasionally dipped into the absurd, once running the 72-mile race around Lake Tahoe. He kept meticulous records of his running. According to a May 4,

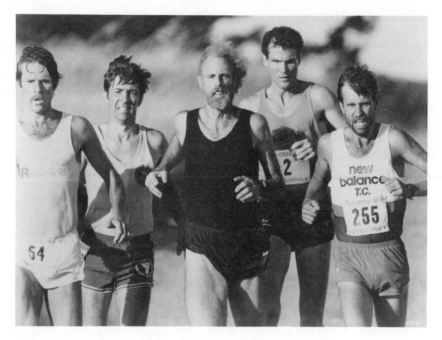

Wes Holman (Bruce Dern, center) breaks through the pack midway through the exhausting, 14-mile Cielo-Sea race, the race he runs at the climax of the film, *On the Edge*. (Photo courtesy of Skouras Pictures)

1986, interview in the *San Francisco Chronicle*, he knew, for instance, that in 26 years of running up to January 17, 1986, when he ran his 100,000th mile, he had missed only 9 days of running. "The rewards still are far greater than the setbacks," he said. "I'm competitive. I don't know what I would do if I couldn't run anymore. I know a lot of people have perished who were addicted to a sport, then couldn't do it anymore" (Zailian, p. 31).

2
CHAPTER

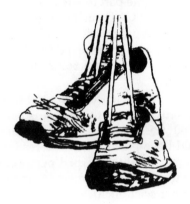

POTENTIAL VICTIM: THE AMATEUR AEROBIC ATHLETE

We live in fascinating times.

People who keep track of such things contend that the store of human knowledge doubles every 10 years. If that is true, a youngster who was 10 years old on January 1, 1989, has seen as much knowledge accumulated in his or her lifetime as was accumulated between the first dawning of a basic truism in protohistoric man (probably something like "Fire burns. Don't touch it.") and December 31, 1979. That's a pretty staggering—and sobering—concept.

All we need do to appreciate the pace of progress is make an inventory of things we already take for granted. Things like VCRs. Ten years ago, how many of us thought that we would soon be able to turn our living room into a movie theater? Even more outrageous: There are more than 2 million satellite dishes in American backyards—satellite dishes that can apprehend signals originating 22,000 miles away in outer space. Not so many decades ago NASA's satellite tracking dishes weren't much more sophisticated—and cost a thousand times as much.

We live in an age of instant communication. A letter that a century ago took 3 months to find its way from New York to Los Angeles can today be faxed 3,000 miles in seconds. Medical advances over the past decade have been enormous, due in large part to advances in technology. Today small-town hospitals are buying CAT scan machines, which a decade ago were confined to only the most progressive—and richest—of the nation's teaching hospitals. The computer has evolved from a multimillion dollar machine that filled two huge rooms to a $69.95 toy that can be carried in a sixth-grader's knapsack.

As a youngster, I used to read science fiction the way a whale gathers plankton: in bushel-basketfuls. Everything that is being realized today was thought of 30 and 40 years ago. One might think that this preview of things to come would have jaded me to the reality of the dream. It hasn't. But it has given me a slightly warped perspective on marvelous things—perhaps because they are less surprising than they are fascinating.

One of the more startling scientific developments of the past decade was the Jarvik-7 artificial heart—now recognized as far from perfect but nonetheless revolutionary when first inserted into a human chest. When the news of the artificial heart hit, my reaction was somewhat left-handed. The device was certainly interesting scientifically, but my response was not, "Look how many lives the artificial heart will save." Considering the millions of Americans who had, during the past decade, taken up an aerobic lifestyle, my response was, "Look at how many people aren't ever going to need that artificial heart!"

In the face of major revolutions brought about by scientific developments (from the industrial revolution to the computer revolution), here was a grass-roots revolution that was going not unnoticed, but somewhat unappreciated.

In the wealthiest, most advanced nation on Earth, where even the modestly affluent could have almost everything done for them instead of doing it themselves, millions of Americans with good educations, good jobs, and good incomes had *chosen* to take control of the physical side of their lives.

They had literally rejected the artificial heart, rejected the advance of science, and had instead *chosen* to do something positive for themselves. In a nation where coronary and related diseases had literally been accepted as the death mode of choice, where for decades the numbers of deaths from heart attack and related causes had spiraled, and where aging ungracefully had become an accepted condition, millions were suddenly saying, "Whoa! Enough is enough. I don't *choose* to accept the inevitable. I don't think rapid aging and heart disease *are* inevitable."

This revolution against traditional lifestyles that not only accepted, but almost encouraged an environment of heart disease did not occur overnight.

THE SIGNIFICANCE OF THE AMATEUR AEROBIC ATHLETE

It would be easy to take the tack of the weekly newsmagazines, which saw fitness as a fad, and say that it emerged in the late 1970s, full-blown, from the post–World War II baby boomer generation.

But actually, as with any revolution, by the time it came to the notice of the average citizen, the "fitness revolution" had had many years to ferment and grow. (See the next section in this chapter, "A Short History of the Amateur Aerobic Athlete.") And, like any other significant revolution, it went well beyond *fad*, used up the term *trend*, and dug itself right into the very fabric of society. The continuing drop in the percentage of Americans dying of heart disease is a significant indicator that the fitness revolution has been building for decades and that it has had a positive effect.

The aerobic fitness revolution is significant on two fronts: It came from the people themselves, and it was so deep-rooted that it persists despite the absence of any unifying organization to promote it. Although, with the huge numbers involved, the fitness revolution can justifiably be called a movement, it is not a movement in the traditional sense because each one taking part does so for personal, individualized reasons, and to no discernible society-changing end other than to feel well and to look good.

This individuality within the greater movement sets it apart from sports-oriented movements of the past. Most of those movements involved team sports that required organizations (softball associations, YMCA or CYO basketball leagues, semipro football teams, and so on) or sports that required a great deal of equipment, a partner or partners, and a place to play (for example, golf and tennis). In addition, many of the past sports movements overlooked more than half the population—women—and even those that did not studiously dragged their feet on allowing females to participate on an equal footing.

No argument could be made that the typical aerobic sport requires a great deal of money, a partner, or a sports arena. It could be argued, however, that aerobic sports *do* have organizations and that they *did* offer resistance to female participation.

On the first count, most aerobic sports participants do not belong to any organization. Runners participating in certain events must buy TAC (The Athletics Congress) memberships, as triathletes need Tri-Fed memberships to take part in some triathletic events. But the memberships are mere formalities to feed the coffers of organizations that had virtually nothing to do with the promotion of the sport to its present importance; the sport grew, in many instances, *in spite* of groups like TAC. In the end, the several organizations for aerobic sports are set in place to regulate the professionals, almost always at the expense of the amateur.

On the issue of female participation, advances in the aerobic sports came quickly by comparison with other sports in this country. In running, the pendulum quickly swung to a situation bordering on reverse discrimination. Women wanted entry in all-men's fields and got it within a relatively few years, while at the same time establishing their own all-women's fields. As a result, there are no longer men-only road races (barring the Olympic men's marathon trials), but there *are* women-only road races.

There is no quick and easy answer as to why, between 1976 and 1986, so many Americans, primarily in their 30s, gave up the sedentary lifestyle and took up the more difficult but infinitely more rewarding endurance lifestyle.

The most romantic idea is that there is a basic need in the human body to move and a basic need in the human psyche to lift us above our technological accomplishments so that we don't get overshadowed by those accomplishments.

Physically speaking, we are made for movement. The largest bones and muscles in the human body are in the legs, and for a very good reason: Because the body was designed to walk, to stride out, to run, to travel. If the body were designed to sit, the biggest muscles would be on the rump, so that this part could handle extended sitting more effectively. As it is, the rump contains the ends of several muscles but is composed almost entirely of fat—fat that tends to spread out when the rump is used too much. In other words, the human body was not designed to get better at sitting the more it sits; the reverse is true. The body rapidly gives in to the dictates of gravity while simultaneously applying great stress to the vertebrae.

The human body was designed the way great inventors can only dream of designing a machine: So that it gets better the more it is used. The typical machine begins to deteriorate with increasing use, as well as with disuse. The human body becomes better and more efficient and stronger the more it is used, so long as it is not abused and is properly maintained.

The cream of the American crop of human beings, the best and the brightest, those who were at the forefront of significant change in the way we live and work and think and communicate, were the ones who responded to the idea that, ''Hey, technology's great, but we need more than this. We need to retain our own personalities, our own selves, throughout these major social changes.''

Many members of the baby boomer generation seemed to want it all: a good education, a good job, a good income, a good body, some physical and psychological fulfillment. By design or by chance, aerobic sports provided the avenue for people who wanted it all to take a giant stride toward their goal. They could have their modern job while stalling aging, while also looking and feeling good, while also getting some personal satisfaction by running, bicycling, taking aerobic dance, swimming, training for and entering triathlons, and so forth. They could rise beyond the concepts of limited horizons: They could be a rocket scientist *and* a 2:45 marathoner, a thinker and a doer.

These millions of Americans in their 30s decided to do rather than to watch someone else do. They were a generation who had been told they could change the world. And, as they aged and faced the overwhelming realities of attempting to change the world, they found that by taking up an aerobic sport they could change, if not the world as a whole, at least their own immediate world. It was a giddy prospect that flew in the face of the generation before them, most of whom had espoused the philosophy that one should work hard for the reward of stopping. When the weekend came for our parents, a fitting reward was to watch paid athletes go head-to-head on television. When retirement came, it was time to stop.

The baby boomers, and some like-minded members of previous generations, saw it otherwise. One worked not with the ultimate goal of stopping, but with the goal of going. The weekend meant the long run or the long bicycle ride in the hills or the citizens' cross-county ski race or the marathon. It wasn't a time to watch other people do something physical, it was a time to *do* something physical: Time to run your own race, not pay to watch other people run theirs.

And the beauty of aerobic sports was that, in most instances, there were no barriers to participation. Whereas a baseball fan couldn't walk into Boston's Fenway Park and play with the Red Sox, but paid merely to watch, an aerobic athlete could pay an entry fee and line up at the same 10K starting line as Frank Shorter or Bill Rodgers, the best in the world.

The difference in concepts, the difference between generations, was significant. And in no time at all another revolutionary idea grown in America would spread all around the world.

A SHORT HISTORY OF THE AMATEUR AEROBIC ATHLETE

It has been said that those who do not know history are doomed to repeat its mistakes. An historical perspective is essential to a full understanding of the many positive and several negative aspects of aerobic sports.

Because walking or running is the simplest of the aerobic pursuits and—excuse the pun—the longest-running, it is appropriate to begin the examination of the aerobic athlete from the perspective of that activity.

As we discussed in the first section of this chapter, the largest bones (the femur in the upper leg) and the largest muscles (the quadriceps or thigh muscles) in the human body are in the legs. The legs also contain the muscles (the calves) with the most densely packed muscle tissue. From primordial times, this concentration of big bones and muscles in the legs helped the human to stand upright (permitting better scanning of surrounding terrain) and promoted walking, striding, jogging, and running as a means of locomotion, thereby increasing the species' effective range.

Before the human became a farmer with a stationary home, the male of the species was a hunter; many of the early human tribes were wanderers or nomads, following the herds that constituted their primary food source. Many Eskimo tribes still cling to this pattern. Primitive man survived as a hunter primarily for three reasons: Because of his brain, he could often outsmart game; if he could not always outsmart it himself, he was capable (again, because of his big brain) of putting together a group of hunters to surround the game; and, if those methods were unsuccessful, the human was quite capable of running his game to death.

Running game to death was fairly common. Falling into what the military used to call a dogtrot (what we now call a jog), the hunter pursued the game until the animal, with its inferior body cooling system, was run to exhaustion and made easy prey.

Even when humans turned to farming as the primary food source, they frequently traveled at a jog pace to visit friends and relatives. Jogging was also necessary for communication: Messengers carrying news and personal correspondence ran between villages. This method of communication was common in a wide variety of cultures.

In Africa, messengers carried a "letter" in the split fork of a stick held aloft. In Hawaii, the king kept in contact with outlying regions and ran the affairs of state using a group of messengers who came to be known as *kykini*, or "the king's messengers." In the Himalayas, messages were (and still are, to some extent) sent by runners between far-flung, high-altitude monasteries. In Greece, communication between city-states was maintained by a group of long-distance runners called *hemerodromoi*, or "all-day runners."

The hemerodromoi carried messages and instructions between different flanks of the Greek armies. The most famous of the wartime hemerodromoi was Pheidippides. Legend has it that after the Athenian victory on the Plains of Marathon, Pheidippides was sent to Athens, just over 20 miles away, to deliver the news. He ran to the steps of Athens, uttered his message, "Nike!", and dropped dead. The legend was merely legend, a bit of romantic drivel created in 1879 by the English poet Robert Browning in his poem to Pheidippides.

In reality, the jaunt from the Plains of Marathon to Athens wasn't much of an exertion for a trained hemerodromos. Several days before the decisive battle, a hemerodromos ran from Athens to Sparta (a distance of 140 miles) to petition assistance, but was refused and had to return the same distance with the distressing news. The runner Pheidippides supposedly made the 140-mile trip to Sparta in less than 36 hours, not an inconceivable accomplishment.

From the days of ancient Greece up to this very century, the military has used runners to deliver messages between points on the battleground. (The film *Gallipoli* is an excellent illustration of this practice.) Runners carried messages through the trenches in World War I.

The accomplishments of military runners notwithstanding, long-distance running has never been regarded with great respect by the sporting public. This may account for the absence of a long-distance running revolution before the 1970s—there wasn't enough money or prestige to be gained from it to interest any but the monetarily independent or the anonymous. In ancient Greece, the incredible accomplishments of the hemerodromoi were taken as a matter of course; after all, that was their job. The laurels in ancient Greece, and ever since then in major running competitions, have always gone to the sprinters.*

The marathon itself came about in the 1896 revival of the Olympic Games as an afterthought in honor of the hosting Greeks. It was an exhibition event, and there were no plans to repeat it. Spiridon Loues, the young Greek who won the first Olympic marathon as the host country's only medalist, assured the preservation of the event, as did a group of New York and Boston fans who came home to the United States and began their own marathons.

Because of the explosion in aerobic athletics over the past decade, we have a slightly distorted view of the prominence of aerobic sports in our century.

At the turn of the century, virtually all competitive running in the United States was done in colleges or athletic clubs (for example, the Boston Athletic Association and the New York Athletic Association, the two groups that supplied most of America's Olympic athletes in 1896). There were a very few practitioners of what we would today think of as ultraendurance sports. Near the turn of the century, there were 24-hour and 6-day endurance events, some for very large purses. The contestants generally walked these events at a brisk pace around a track, often indoors, while spectators bet on the outcome.

---

*In the first 13 ancient Olympics for which records are extant, there was only one event contested: a sprint race one length of the stadium, or about 200 yards. Other events were added as the ancient Olympics matured and later deteriorated under Roman rule.

General physical fitness was mostly confined to rudimentary programs in private schools and some compulsory exercise as part of the regimen in the military. Training theories relative to running were insane by today's standards: For example, a high-school miler would be told never to run a mile in practice because it would exhaust him in advance of the competition; the miler was thus limited to running a half mile at a time, and on occasion a 3/4 mile, but never the distance of the event itself, and certainly never *beyond* the distance to be contested.

The depression era saw considerable interest in marathon-type events— specifically, marathon dance contests and several editions of a cross-the-country endurance running contest known as the Bunion Derby—but the events were more spectacle than sport, a way to divert attention from the extreme conditions in a country that had had the pins knocked out from under it.

The late 1930s and the 1940s saw some interest in physical fitness generated by pioneers like Jack LaLanne, who developed his "physical culture" studios.

The first public emphasis on general physical fitness in recent times came during the John F. Kennedy administration. This push took the form of the then-famous 50-mile walks, a response to the news that Russians were more fit than Americans and that American children were lagging behind Russian children in education. (In the media, a mythical American youngster named Johnny was compared with Ivan, his Russian counterpart.)

The Kennedy legacy, in part due to JFK's charisma, was one of increased awareness of physical education in the schools (which has since fallen off drastically) and, for a small percentage of the population, a regular pursuit of physical fitness for its own sake.

The next great ripple in the physical fitness Sea of Tranquility came in 1968 with the publication of *Aerobics*. Dr. Kenneth Cooper had developed his program while a doctor in the air force. On the basis of research available at the time, Cooper concluded that by raising the heart rate through moderate exercise for 20 minutes three or four times a week, a person could lower the risk of heart disease, improve weight control, and generally feel better and more capable physically.

Cooper's book came at a propitious moment. Death by heart-related diseases had climbed at an alarming rate. Cardiac disorder had become the fatal disease of choice in the United States. A goodly number of intelligent businessmen who were approaching the age when an American male could expect to develop heart problems discovered Cooper's book, adopted his program, and began to feel and look better than they had in years. In a manner not unlike a pyramid selling scheme, an executive won over to the program began preaching the aerobic doctrine to any peer who would listen, and the book, although published by one of the smaller firms, gained tremendous word-of-mouth support.

At the heart of the aerobics program was jogging, the easiest form of strenuous aerobic exercise available. The simplicity of a jogging program appealed to the busy executive: It required no investment of time to learn a new skill; it was easy to schedule into a busy day; it required no special facilities, no partner or team, and minimal equipment, so it tended to travel well. Upcoming executives in major companies, who saw their superiors jogging and decided that it might have had something to do with their success, took up the sport as well. Since Cooper encouraged people to jog at a speed comfortable enough to permit talking, executives found themselves holding informal meetings on the run. For the executive who was already into another sport like golf or tennis, jogging had the added benefit of building endurance in the legs and increasing one's "wind" (cardiovascular endurance).

Cooper's program specified 20-minute workouts. These 20 minutes were long enough to bestow a cardiovascular benefit and were short enough to fit nicely into a tight schedule.

The deviates from Cooper's program—those who went beyond the prescribed 20 minutes—began to enter and run in road races that were usually put on by small local running clubs. These new runners began swelling the rather meager ranks of the long-distance running community in the United States, until then almost invisible. As a result, the clubs began holding more and more races to take advantage of the growing interest in their previously arcane sport.

Following the 1972 Olympic Games, there was increased participation in Olympic sports in general, and in endurance events in particular. This phenomenon was not unique. The year following an Olympics traditionally saw increased interest in the sports that the games highlighted. Increased—and more sophisticated—television coverage of the Olympics brought the inspiring performances into an ever-larger number of American homes and in turn inspired more and more people to take up one or another sport that was showcased in the games.

One of the most inspiring performances in the 1972 Olympics was Frank Shorter literally running away from a group of the best distance runners in the world.

In this performance, Shorter, a member of the baby boom generation, inspired hundreds of thousands of his fellow boomers to take up running. He also inspired thousands of Americans already running on Cooper's aerobics program to increase their weekly distances. And the lure of running the marathon suddenly hung in the air. Business executives, used to taking on and methodically surmounting challenges in the business world, applied their talents to training for and running a marathon.

Boomers, brought up on the philosophy that anything is possible, suddenly wanted to do what Shorter had done.

By the time the 1976 Olympic Games in Montreal came along, America was primed to explode into what has come to be known as the *running revolution*.

Participation in marathons in the United States increased. In response, running clubs put together more marathons to accommodate the increased interest.

Let's take a moment to examine this trend. What follows are runner participation figures for some sample years in the Boston Marathon, the world's oldest continuously run marathon:

> 1898—21 runners
> 1928—254 runners
> 1964—300 runners
> 1967—600 runners
> 1969—1,150 runners
> 1970—1,011 runners*
> 1973—1,384 runners**
> 1974—1,705 runners
> 1975—2,090 runners
> 1976—1,898 runners***
> 1977—3,000 runners
> 1978—6,000 runners
> 1979—7,800 runners
> 1980—5,400 runners****
> 1981—7,000 runners

BENEFITS OF THE AEROBIC LIFESTYLE

Considering the benefits derived from an aerobic lifestyle, it is not surprising that millions of highly educated Americans concerned with maintaining a youthful appearance and feeling better physically took up aerobic exercise.

To appreciate the physical and psychological benefits of a regular aerobic program, let us take time to review those benefits. An appreciation of the many potential benefits will later put into perspective some

---

* 4:00 qualifying time instituted; ** 3:30 qualifying time put into place; *** 3:00 qualifying time in effect; **** 2:50 qualifying time used.

athletes' tendency to persist in aerobic activities even at the risk of physical and emotional injury.

An increasing number of studies conducted on adults who exercise aerobically on a regular basis indicate that such exercise offers a battery of benefits.

For instance, a recent study by Kasch, Wallace, Van Camp, and Verity (1988) and associates titled "A Longitudinal Study of Cardiovascular Stability in Active Men Aged 45 to 65 Years" concerned 15 men who exercised aerobically—walking, running, swimming, bicycling—an average of 3.6 days a week for 20 years, expending 2,104 kilocalories per week on average. The study found that their VO_2max (a measure of aerobic work efficiency) declined only 12 percent over those 20 years, as opposed to an anticipated decline of 1 to 2 percent per year, or 20 to 40 percent.

In a two-part round-table discussion on the health benefits of exercise (Rippe, 1987a, 1987b), prominent experts enumerated these benefits, as derived from 40 major studies conducted on the topic over the past 25 years: cardiovascular improvement, metabolic benefits, weight loss, a possible decrease in cancer risk, lowered risk of osteoporosis, greater physical work capacity, increased cardiac output, lower blood pressure, and reduced incidence of hypertension. Unfortunately, the panel lamented, fewer than 20 percent of adult Americans exercise regularly enough to reap these benefits.

Let's take a closer look at the major benefits of a regular aerobic sports program.

Physical Benefits

1. *Promotes cardiovascular health.* First and foremost to benefit from regular aerobic exercise are the heart and the circulatory system. The heart is a muscle much like other muscles in the body. If it is exercised, it becomes stronger and, to a degree, larger. If it it *not* used regularly, it loses tone and efficiency; it becomes weak, and as the body needs its services more and more, it is less and less able to deliver the goods. So, regular aerobic exercise that causes the heart muscle to work at a higher level— but not an *excessively* high level—and maintain that level for 20 to 30 minutes three or four times a week builds up the heart's ability to do its job.

Additionally, aerobic exercise improves the circulatory system by expanding its ability to carry oxygen- and nutrient-rich blood through the body's intricate system of arteries and vessels. Such exercise also increases the amount of high-density lipoproteins (HDL) in the blood, thereby contributing to a more favorable serum cholesterol level; HDL has been found to remove damaging low-density lipoproteins (LDL) and very low-density lipoproteins (VLDL) from the bloodstream, helping the fight against arteriosclerosis. (For more information, see "Fitness, Heart Disease, and High-Density Lipoproteins: A Look at the Relationships," McCunney, 1987.)

2. *Improves muscle tone.* The activity that causes the heart to exercise systematically uses major muscle groups in a repetitive manner. It is the working requirements of these muscle groups that trigger the heart to pump more blood to provide needed oxygen and nutrients to allow the muscle groups to continue functioning. As the muscles cause the heart to work on their behalf, they are also doing primary work, which increases their own strength and efficiency, allowing them to function well under additional loads. This in turn builds muscle tone. The working muscles, by doing what they were created to do, get better at doing it (unlike machines of metal and plastic, which wear out with use). Using the muscles aerobically adds strength and efficiency *without* necessarily adding a great deal of bulk.

3. *Increases energy stores.* Efficient, toned muscles work better than inefficient, untoned muscles. A by-product of this added efficiency is that the regularly working muscles amass a great deal of *potential* energy. The concept of a "lean, mean fighting machine" is appropriate when applied to muscles made fit and toned by regular aerobic exercise. A toned muscle is capable of delivering work readily through both efficiency of motion and additional energy stores not available in an inefficient muscle. The motto here is: Energy begets energy.

4. *Lowers body fat.* A well-toned muscle group becomes aesthetically attractive by gradually metabolizing unnecessary body fat stores. The lean machine has no need or use for a great deal of stored fatty tissue. As a person engages in an aerobic program, the body is fueled by calories provided by food taken in or by fat stored in the body. Typically, at the outset of a fitness program, the body quickly learns to use both food *and* stored fat. Little by little, the regular activity cuts more and more into the fat stores and burns them, causing a loss of body fat while there is a corresponding increase in muscle mass. Muscle weighs more than fat because it is more dense, but muscle tissue consumes less space. This is why the person who has recently embarked on a fitness program sometimes weighs as much as, or more than, he or she did before starting the program. Fat is being burned, and muscle fibers enlarge to accommodate the ever-increasing capacity of energy-producing processes within. For this reason it is best to forget weighing yourself when beginning a fitness program; the scale often gives a distorted picture of what is happening to your body. Measurement of selected body parts is a much more accurate monitoring device.

5. *Slows the resting pulse rate.* Besides building up certain body systems, making the human machine more efficient also slows down other

functions. Aerobic exercise builds up the heart, making it a more efficient pump with an increased capacity to pump blood on a given stroke. This capacity is referred to as stroke volume. As stroke volume is increased, the heart can meet the body's needs with fewer strokes. These strokes are measured in the pulse rate. The more efficient the heart, the fewer beats per minute are necessary to meet the body's needs.

6. *Lowers blood pressure.* As aerobic exercise increases the flexibility and the potential volume of the system of arteries and vessels, and as the exercise promotes the HDL that clear the interior walls of the arteries, less force is needed to move the life-giving blood through the vascular system; the result is lower blood pressure.

7. *Lowers cholesterol.* The greatest cause of heart disease in this country is less a weakening of the heart than a weakening of the major blood vessels or a closure of those vessels by cholesterol-created plaque, accounting for arteriosclerosis, or hardening of the arteries. A reduction in blood cholesterol has been shown to result from regular aerobic exercise done in concert with dietary modifications that lower overall cholesterol intake. If you lower cholesterol, the chances of heart disease are significantly lowered as well.

8. *Relieves muscular stress.* Regular aerobic exercise has also been shown to reduce muscular stress caused by everyday psychological stress that may originate with tense situations, but that often manifests itself in physical muscle tension, especially in the neck, shoulders, and lower back.

9. *Promotes restorative sleep.* Regular aerobic exercise *does* cause the body to become blissfully weary. The physical demands of exercise tire the muscles, which require rest to rebuild themselves and come back stronger. This need for rest has a delightful side effect for people who, with age, find it more and more difficult to get a good night's sleep. Regular exercise tends to promote sleep by physically tiring the body. Many people taking up an aerobic exercise program are pleasantly astonished at the quality and quantity of sleep they get.

10. *Promotes regularity of bowel movements.* Another side effect of regular aerobic exercise is the promotion of digestive regularity. With the typical American low-fiber diet, irregularity becomes more of a problem as we age. Regular exercise assists the body in moving food through the digestive system and in evacuating waste.

Psychological Benefits

1. *Builds self-esteem.* It is easy to imagine the tremendous improvement in self-esteem of a person who has been nonathletic for the first 35 years of life and who then takes up, for instance, long-distance running and

within 3 or 4 years successfully runs a marathon. Frequently, the amateur aerobic athete was not an athlete in high school or college, was never picked for sandlot teams, was possibly never chosen for stickball at recess in grade school. Now, he or she is one of fewer than 200,000 people (in a country of 242,000,000) who last year completed a marathon. The runner's self-esteem can't help but skyrocket. The phenomenon has been repeated millions of times over the last decade as non-athletes took up an aerobic sport, became comfortable with it, and continued to push farther. And these people did not have to go from chronic nonathlete to marathoner to do it. Increased self-esteem can come from moving, over a 5-year period, from being a nonathlete to training for and successfully completing a 10K road race in under an hour. Self-esteem can also result from physical changes brought about by participation in aerobic activity. A 30-year-old woman, overfat for the past 10 years, who takes up aerobic dancing and builds muscle tissue while burning body fat is likely to raise her self-esteem significantly as she reshapes her body. And this rise in self-esteem engendered by success in a fitness program will have positive spillover consequences in her personal life.

2. *Promotes psychological release.* For amateur athletes who are not obsessive in their training, running, swimming, or bicycling an hour each day can serve as a better safety valve and psychological outlet than a 2-hour session with a psychiatrist. To quote Doug Latimer, the former publisher of *Women's Sports and Fitness* and the Western States 100 champion: "Running has been a great relief from stress. Starting this magazine and running it for 9 years has been one pressure after another. We are underfinanced all the way. I can't remember how many times I have woken up in the middle of the night and not been able to go back to sleep because next day was payroll and we had to pay the print bill and there was no way in the world we were going to be able to do it. We always did, though. Things are going well for me right now; but it was tough, and without running I think I would have had a heart attack, cancer, I might have had a mental breakdown, might have gotten divorced, just no telling. But being able to go out and run at lunch time for 45 minutes or after work for an hour made a big difference."

3. *Promotes a sense of well-being and equanimity.* Feelings of well-being and equanimity are psychological cornerstones of endurance training—and racing. The sense of well-being springs directly from the physical side of training; regular training, occasionally spiced with extraordinarily fine workouts, creates a feeling of accomplishment and satisfaction and a fine pool of well-being into which the amateur athlete can sink. The involvement also produces a sense of equanimity, especially for older participants who came to endurance sports well beyond the age of college

athletics. Such a person had every reason to believe that his or her athletic career—and therefore a sense of his or her physical self—was over. The satisfaction of finding a new athletic environment that offers continued opportunity to train and compete, and in which the physical side of life is anything but over, fosters a sense of peace and rightness that descends like a mantle over the person.

4. *Promotes sociability and camaraderie.* A silly theory about runners was espoused well before the running revolution; it contended that long-distance runners were introverted, that introverts gravitated to long-distance running. According to the theory, since so much distance running was done solo, there was only one psychological profile that needed apply. That *may* have been true of long-distance runners before the running revolution, but it hasn't been true since 1978. A lot of silence occurs just before a race, as the runners stretch, loosen up, jog a bit to get the early-morning tightness out of the legs, and attempt to get psychologically "up" for the coming event. After the race, however, the finish area is like the Tower of Babel, with runners chattering and comparing notes, making introductions and rerunning the race. In many races, conversation fills the early miles while the runners still have enough oxygen to talk.

Camaraderie among endurance athletes extends to one and all, perhaps in part because endurance sports foster mass participation; Joe Schmo can run with and against Bill Rodgers in the same event; Joe Blow can enter a triathlon and compete against Dave Scott. Sharing territory and experiences—the race course, the temperature—tumbles barriers and forms common ground.

5. *Encourages setting and achieving of goals.* Very few amateur athletes take up an endurance sport with a whole set of short- and long-term goals formulated. Most amateurs dabble at their sport initially, often merely to get into better shape. Their goals are somewhat amorphous: They want to drop a few pounds, get their wind back, fit into their clothes a little better, look a little better overall, hold back the onslaught of time. They seldom have specific short-term goals, much less long-term goals, unless you count the number of aerobic points they hope to achieve each week. For most neophyte amateur endurance athletes, however, the matter of short-term and long-term goal setting emerges with more thorough involvement in the sport. The goal-setting process can bring order to their lives, and often has positive carryover effects outside of sport. Successful attainment of goals also strengthens their belief that they can apply the same determination to other aspects of life.

6. *Promotes a healthy competitive nature.* The late bloomer in aerobic sports who trains hard to compete in an event frequently kindles a competitive spark in the psyche. It is astonishing, in some instances, to see

the transformation that takes place when a usually sensitive, reserved, mild-mannered person engages in competition. When the starter's gun fires, such people become incredibly competitive, and when the race is finished, they revert to their former shy, retiring selves. It is almost as though, denied the physical outlet for 25, 30, or more years, they are making up for lost time by releasing stored-up (and fermented) competitive juices. Many thrive on it, and some become so motivated that they become quite good at their sport. Certainly, most endurance sports are not contact sports and therefore do not require a massive physique; in fact, they favor the lean over the massive. In these sports the former shy and retiring person of modest stature can find an arena in which not only to compete, but in which to actually excel. Some of this newfound competitiveness can spill over into the person's everyday life in a very positive way.

COOPER VERSUS SHORTER: HEALTH VERSUS SATISFACTION

As previously discussed, a regular program of aerobic exercise as prescribed by Cooper (20 minutes three or four times a week) brings a multitude of benefits, both physical and psychological.

This knowledge became so commonplace during the running and fitness revolution that an axiom of George Sheehan—running's guru—was developed and disseminated freely to anyone who would listen: "The first 20 minutes of aerobic exercise is for your body—anything beyond is for yourself."

The quote, ironically, came not from those pushing the 20 minutes of exercise, but from those who had pushed well beyond it: those who preferred not to walk in the footsteps of Cooper but to run in pursuit of the footprints of Frank Shorter. It was, to many, not a case of ignoring Cooper's wisdom and accepting the quest for the perfect run that Shorter represented, it was actually the best of both worlds.

By running or doing other aerobic exercise for 45 minutes to an hour or more, an amateur athlete was accepting Cooper's teachings (at least for the first 20 minutes) and was also indulging the quest to become a better athlete. In essence, the first 20 minutes brought the bulk of the physical benefits, while everything beyond piled up the psychological benefits.

Some who ran down the aerobic aisle were of the more-is-always-better school, certainly: people who felt that bigger is better, that if 20 minutes is good, 60 minutes is three times as good.

This philosophy, unfortunately, does not necessarily apply to aerobic exercise.

Although his original theories are now over 20 years old, Cooper's prescription of three or four 20-minute sessions per week has held up fairly well. Nearly 20 years after the publication of Cooper's *Aerobics* in 1968, Ralph Paffenbarger, the force behind the incredible (and massive) ongoing Harvard alumni study, found that an expenditure of 2,000 or more kilocalories per week (to a limit of 3,500 kilocalories per week) of exercise lowered mortality rates by one quarter to one third.

The Harvard alumni study is one of the most ambitious epidemiological studies in the world. For decades, Paffenbarger (1986) and his colleagues have been following the lifestyles of Harvard University alumni. The study involves people between the ages of 35 and 74; at the time of research dealing with benefits of exercise for longevity, it included 16,936 subjects. The longevity research centered on 1,413 alumni who had died between 1962 and 1978.

To quote from the abstract of the study:

Exercise reported as walking, stair climbing, and sports play related inversely to total mortality, primarily to death due to cardiovascular or respiratory causes. Death rates declined steadily as energy expended on such activity increased from less than 500 to 3500 kcal [kilocalories] per week, beyond which rates increased slightly. (Paffenbarger, 1986, p. 605)

The conclusion was that very moderate exercise can add 1 to 2 years of life in a typical 80-year lifetime.

Since 20 minutes of exercise (in this instance jogging at an 8-minute mile) four times a week accounts for 10 miles of jogging per week, this translates for a 150-pound male into an exercise expenditure of about 1,280 kilocalories per week. Dial in the fact that (as recent research has indicated) regular aerobic exercise raises the metabolism and keeps it up for more than 12 hours after the exercise is completed, and our typical follower of Cooper's program is burning roughly 2,000 to 2,500 kilocalories per week. This puts him or her into the life extension category of the Harvard study.

But what about those who go beyond Cooper's limits? What happens to them?

To begin, let's briefly examine some of the physiology that occurs with Cooper's subjects.

First of all, let's admit that 80 minutes out of 10,080 possible minutes in a week (that's four 20-minute exercise sessions per week) is not a staggering investment of time and effort if one is to realize all of the physical benefits we discussed in the last section of this chapter. Most people spend more time than that commuting to work 5 days a week—lots more.

Let's also admit, however, that only a very small percentage of Americans in 1968 were willing to invest 80 minutes a week toward protection against heart disease, weight control, lower blood pressure, lower pulse rate, better muscle tone, regularity, and so on. And the majority of those willing to make that investment were middle-aged, professional males: men who had been willing, during their business lives, to weigh the facts, consider the options, and then make the investment that seemed most advantageous. They were also the Americans in the high-risk group for heart attacks: male and middle-aged, with a fair degree of stress in their lives. These men were, literally, waiting for someone like Cooper to come along with an offer they couldn't logically refuse. They consequently did not ask whether what they were going to be doing would be fun, whether it would be enjoyable. Their question was: In the end, will it help me? If it will, I'll do it.

They did it, and it helped. The enjoyment they derived from their 20-minute jogging sessions came not from the exercise itself, but from the end results of that exercise. They looked better, they felt better, they functioned better physically and mentally. They didn't necessarily enjoy the jogging, but hey, it was a 20-minute investment in their future, and what's 20 minutes out of 1,440 minutes in a day, even for a busy executive?

From a physiological standpoint, what happened in 20 minutes? Quite a bit that would add to the physical health of the executives, but very little that was pleasant.

As we mentioned previously, the word *aerobic* means with oxygen. Its converse is *anaerobic*, or without oxygen.

A marathoner at mile 5 of a 26-mile marathon is typically running aerobically: He or she is running relaxed, breathing rhythmically, and able to chat with a partner while continuing to run. Anaerobic is a sprinter doing a 100-meter dash: The breathing is a series of gasps; the exercise is outstripping the body's ability to take in and transport oxygen to the runner's muscles, expecially those huge leg muscles. The last thing a sprinter can do is chat with the sprinter in the next lane as they go shooting past the 50-meter mark. In anaerobic exercise, the oxygen coming from the lungs is inadequate to feed the muscles; some of the muscle needs are fulfilled by chemical processes deep within the muscles and must be paid for after the activity is finished.

A person embarking on an aerobic exercise session experiences anaerobic exercise at first because she or he is going from a quiet state to a relatively active state. The body's first response is to go anaerobic to meet the sudden increase in oxygen demand indicated by the now-moving muscles. This is why the breathing during the first minutes of aerobic exercise is so noticeable. Aerobic exercise starts anaerobically until the body recognizes that the oxygen needs of the muscles are being adequately filled. Depending on one's state of fitness, this minor oxygen debt can take anywhere from a few minutes to 10 minutes to be met. As soon as it is met, the breathing settles in and the exercising switches to aerobic. This changeover is typically considered the second wind. (This is why top marathoners warm up before starting a race: to change over from anaerobic to aerobic before the race begins and to get the leg muscles loosened.)

Those first 5 to 10 minutes of exercise are not very pleasant. The body is shifting all sorts of gears, building itself to adequately handle what is to come. Getting the huge leg muscles warmed up all the way down into the heart of the muscle, deep inside that closely-packed tissue, takes even longer.

In reality, a human body that exercises for 20 minutes is literally working inefficiently, and the experience is not very pleasant.

However, depending on the individual body, there is a point somewhere between 30 and 40 minutes into aerobic exercise when the breathing settles in and the muscles warm up. The stride becomes smoother; the breathing is almost as natural as when the person is sitting around watching television; the muscles have warmed up; and any little aches and pains have vanished because of the massaging effect of the warmed muscles and the release by the brain of endorphins, natural opiate-like chemicals that mediate minor aches and that lift the athlete's spirit. (This point was noted by both Glasser and Kostrubala in their landmark books.)

That 30- to 40-minute point is the no-man's-land that divides Cooper's disciples from Shorter's followers. It is a point beyond which the exercise becomes anything but drudgery. It is also the reason that many people who have taken up running and other aerobic activities find the sports boring: They have never gone beyond 20 minutes into the region where, on certain days, the effort can become almost effortless.

Whereas exercising under 20 minutes offers no real intrinsic lures but is done as a means to an end, exercising beyond 40 minutes takes on a number of attractions. Below 20 minutes, exercising tends to be boring; beyond 40 minutes, it can become pleasurable. For many, aerobic exercise beyond 40 minutes is a place that serves as a safe harbor from stress and adversity. It is also, as we shall see later, a place where each extra minute has its own charm and where there is always the urge to do more.

For those who go too far too fast, it is also a place that holds an increased risk of exercise-related injuries, which may account for the fact that in the Harvard study, the good effects begin to pale slightly beyond the 3,500-kilocalories-per-week expenditure (for a runner, about 30 miles a week). The good effects may be offset by injuries and other problems.

There is no doubt, however, that the region beyond 40 minutes is the realm of the serious amateur aerobic athlete.

THE SERIOUS AMATEUR VERSUS THE PRO

Occasionally, the professional aerobic athlete is stricken with addiction to workouts or races. The total number of professionals is too small, however, to have significant impact on the primary discussions of this book. Moreover, the professionals in the sport who succumb to abject addiction to their workouts and races are likely to find that they aren't professionals for long. One characteristic of addiction is an inability to judge when dedication to working out goes overboard to the point that it negatively affects performance; this decided tendency to overtrain would undercut a professional's effort to realize his or her potential.

For clarity, let us define professional aerobic athletes as those who earn more than half of their income from the sport. Typically, the professional athlete is paid to compete in a race and is also eligible for prize money based upon performance. The pro may also earn money promoting a product (endorsing Oakley sunglasses, running for and endorsing a specific shoe company's product, and so forth) or selling a product, typically activewear, that bears his or her name linked with a competitive reputation.

An aerobic athlete who sells shoes 30 hours a week at an athletic shoe store and who occasionally wins a couple of dollars in a race is not a professional in this context, since the majority of the person's income is earned in the shoe salesperson's job. Nor can an amateur aerobic athlete who regularly competes in races and occasionally wins money for doing so be considered professional.

Bill Rodgers, in contrast, is a professional. He is paid handsomely for appearing at races and for placing well in them, he has his name on a line of running apparel and is paid a percentage of sales, and he owns two running stores that bear his name.

But Brad Hawthorne of Oakland, California, who at this point in his life can run a marathon faster than Rodgers, is not a professional runner, even though he has won several thousand dollars at the Big Sur International Marathon and the Las Vegas International Marathon. He is a full-time management-level employee of the Chevron Oil Company, and he makes his living from working at Chevron, not from running.

Although it is relatively easy to draw a line between the professional aerobic athlete and the top-level serious amateur aerobic athlete, it is harder to draw a line below the serious amateur—a line that would divide the serious from the average amateur aerobic athlete.

We have indicated that the upper limit for the Cooper–inspired athlete is 20 minutes a day, three to four days a week. This athlete need never be concerned with worrying about the next exercise fix.

But where is the line that separates the serious amateur from the casual amateur?

It is fairly easy to draw an approximate borderline that separates the physically serious from the not-so-serious. The borderline would not be very wide, and it would read something like this:*

> Running—25 to 30 miles per week
> Swimming—5 to 7 miles per week
> Cycling—75 to 100 miles per week
> Aerobic dance—3 to 4 hours per week

The distance and time standards of such a borderline might be met by even a casual aerobic athlete on occasion throughout the year, often in preparation for an annual competitive event. This does not make the athlete a serious amateur, however. To fall in the serious category, one must consistently meet or exceed the borderline standards.

A better indication of seriousness is a typical weekly work level that reflects these minimum standards, along with an *attitude*, which is more difficult to measure. How important to the athlete's overall lifestyle is the ritual of workout, the necessity of racing? How much of that lifestyle is dictated by the chosen aerobic sport?

Although it is difficult to lay firm ground rules about attitude, there is little doubt when one is talking with a person who is a serious amateur, and probably less doubt when that person has passed over the line into addiction.

For this discussion, a serious amateur athlete regularly meets the borderline requirements indicated above (or comparable measures for other aerobic sports) and is sufficiently involved in the sport that it noticeably influences his or her general lifestyle (see self-test, next page).

THE THREE TYPES OF AMATEUR AEROBIC ATHLETES

To better understand the aerobic athlete and the problems that can be encountered in a serious aerobic lifestyle, let us separate the millions of serious aerobic athletes into three categories on the basis of the athletic background—or lack of same—from which they came.

---

*It is impossible to create such a borderline for multisport athletes, since a triathlete's emphasis on each of the three sports varies widely throughout the training regimen. In such a case it is usually easiest to create a borderline by counting hours per week dedicated to workouts, excluding time spent changing clothes between sports, showering, and other such activities. That range would be 5 to 8 hours per week.

A Self-Test
How Serious an Amateur Athlete Are You?

Place an X in front of each of the following statements that applies to you and your endurance fitness. Then, total your Xs and see the interpretations at the end of this test.

_____ During most weeks of the year, I tend to train and/or race 5 or more days.

_____ At least two of my workouts in a typical week are 60 minutes or longer.

_____ I occasionally or regularly do double workouts (two workouts in one day).

_____ The most serene times I experience in the typical week are those times I spend exercising alone.

_____ I occasionally or regularly do a long workout of 2 or more hours.

_____ In a typical year, I race/compete a dozen times or more.

_____ I occasionally or regularly have sleepless nights for no apparent reason.

_____ My regular aerobic workouts are an important means of stress release for me.

_____ If I were independently wealthy, I could afford to put as much time into my training as I currently put into my full-time job or occupation.

_____ I tend to know more about the latest performances of the top professional athletes in my aerobic sport than I know the candidates and issues in national elections.

_____ There is no doubt in my mind that the world would be a better place if more people participated in aerobic sports.

_____ Socially, I tend to gravitate toward fellow athletes.

_____ Since I have taken up an aerobic lifestyle, my life in general has become more well rounded.

_____ I have found it necessary on occasion to train through an injury; if I have never had an injury, I feel I would tend to train through it.

_____ My diet has changed since I have taken up an aerobic lifestyle: I tend to gravitate toward healthy foods.

_____ TOTAL YOUR SCORE.

How serious an aerobic athlete are you? 13-15, extremely serious; 10-12, very serious; 7-9, serious amateur; 4-6, moderately serious; 0-3 Ken Cooper devotee.

The classic pyramid graph illustrates this scheme of categories. The pyramid houses every one of the millions of people currently pursuing an aerobic sport at a serious level.

At the top of the pyramid are the professional aerobic athletes: for example, Frank Shorter, Bill Rodgers, Ed Eyestone, Pat Porter, and Joan Benoit Samuelson in long-distance running; Greg LeMonde and John Howard in bicycling; Dave Scott, Kirsten Hanssen, and Scott Tinsley in the triathlon. The top of the pyramid contains a very small percentage of all the serious aerobic athletes, but it contains the best of the breed—or at least the best who have decided to make a living from the sport. They are, in essence, supported by the three larger groups below them. By that I mean that the professionals would not be making their present incomes were it not for the mass of amateur aerobic athletes involved in the sport. Entry fees of the masses contribute to the prize money the pros pick up; the favorable demographics of the involved masses are what draws the sponsors, who in turn put up prize money for the pros; and a percentage of the purchase price of each pair of running shoes, each bicycle, each pair of Oakley sunglasses that the masses buy helps pay for the pros' endorsements.

The three groups of serious aerobic athletes that make up the mass of the aerobic pyramid are as follows:

1. Returning endurance athletes
2. Crossover athletes
3. Nonathletes

Let's take a moment to examine each of these three categories.

The Pyramid of Endurance Athletes

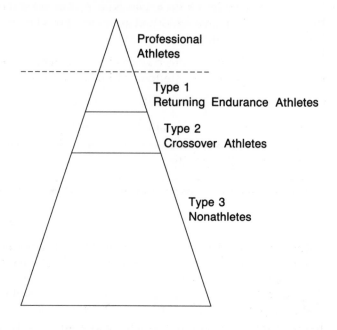

Type 1: Returning Endurance Athletes

The group of returning endurance athletes is larger than the professional group, but not nearly as large as the crossover or the nonathlete group.

It is not very large simply because there were—and are—very few forums in which a young person could be an aerobic athlete in high school or college. The triathlon had not yet been invented in 1972; there were certainly no triathlon teams in high school or college, and there are still precious few (although that likely will change). This pattern extends to other aerobic sports. Between 1978 and 1980, Paul Asmuth, the world's foremost endurance swimmer, was a three-time All-American in the 1,650-yard freestyle (1,500 meters in Olympic and international competition) while attending Arizona State. The 1,650 freestyle was and still is the longest event in competition. Asmuth only glimpsed his true place in swimming history when he took part in 5,000-meter time trials that were part of the training regimen. He found that the farther up he moved, the farther behind his competition fell.

Most of the sports that are part of high school and college life are the typical ball sports: football, basketball, and baseball. None are aerobic sports, although basketball *can* border on aerobics when the game's tempo is picked up and then maintained, in the face of interruptions for timeouts, foul shots, and jump balls. Many schools offer track and field, but the only events that encourage aerobic-style training are the longer running events: 880 yards/800 meters, mile/1,500 meters, and 2 miles.

Although not prevalent in most high schools and colleges, soccer, lacrosse, and field hockey are sports that tend to be marginally aerobic, not so much for the way they are played as for the type of endurance training (primarily running) they demand.

The closest to a high school or college aerobic athlete one can find is the cross-country runner, but cross-country is a minor sport at most schools in this country, and the typical team consists of fewer than a dozen athletes.

Still, the number of high school and college aerobic athletes who ceased training upon graduation, then later in life returned to their high school or college aerobic sport—the returning athletes—accounts for more aerobic athletes than there are professionals. It is also the group that frequently contributes members to that rank who are not quite professionals but are top regional competitors, and who usually continued to pursue their sport (frequently running) after graduation.

Type 2: Crossover Athletes

Because of the number of high school and college-age people who could be accommodated by the major scholastic sports (again, football, basketball, and baseball), there was a vast pool of former nonaerobic athletes who saw the encroaching signs of aging such as unwanted adipose tissue, decided to do something about it, and jumped on the aerobic bandwagon as it began to roll.

These athletes in many cases welcomed the running and fitness revolution because most of them had felt that the ending of their scholastic sports careers meant the end of their sports involvement, outside of the occasional softball league or the company bowling team. In many instances, the only way they could hope to stay involved with the sport they had loved was to coach youngsters in that sport.

The aerobic revolution offered not only a diversion but a real catharsis for many of these people. They were given another lease on their athletic lives, and many took to aerobic sports with great enthusiasm, even if they didn't happen to be genetically predisposed to endurance-type activities.

A distance runner, for example, needs long, lean muscles capable of lengthy effort, in contrast to the football linebacker's heavy blocks of muscle capable of explosive performance. Although a person is genetically predisposed to one muscle type or the other, the human body is an adaptive machine. Alan Page played professional football for 15 years, first with the Minnesota Vikings and then with the Chicago Bears. He was the first lineman in history to win the National Football League's most valuable player award. In 1977 he began running; he weighed 250 pounds and stood 6 feet, 3-1/4 inches. After several years of involvement in long-distance running, he came down to 215 pounds and managed to break 40 minutes in the 10K, a notable performance.

The irony for the crossover category is that, while the athlete was a member of the football or basketball or baseball team, running laps was a punishment imposed by the coach. If a player spoke out of turn or goofed up on a play routine, he was told, "Take a lap!" To many former ball players who crossed over to aerobic sports, taking a lap suddenly felt like the best thing they could possibly do for themselves.

Type 3: Nonathletes

Nonathletes make up by far the largest category of the aerobic pyramid.

Nonathletes are people who either never went out for organized sports or, when they did, did not make the team. In a school of 1,000 students, with perhaps 40 spots open on the football team, 20 on the baseball team, and a dozen on the basketball team, and with some students lettering in more than one sport, nonathletes make up well over 90 percent of the student body.

For many of these people, who felt inadequate for team sports in high school or college, the aerobic sports—which acknowledge individuality, stress perseverance over raw talent, are usually noncontact, and are open to everyone—came as a godsend. An aerobic athlete doesn't have to compete at all.

The scrawny 30-year-old accountant who never made a sports team may find himself at an advantage over the lumbering football lineman when he takes up long-distance running. And the skill requirements for running are almost nonexistent, the sport is so basic and simple.

For the nonathlete, the aerobic revolution was like being handed a second childhood—just at a time in life when a second childhood would serve a better purpose than three sessions a week with a psychologist.

Amateur aerobic athletes in all three classes, then, have reasons to be grateful for the aerobic revolution:

• Type 1—The *returning endurance athlete,* rediscovering a sport she or he enjoyed in younger times, finds it just as enjoyable if not more so, because now it can be done individually instead of under the pressure associated with a team.

• Type 2—The *cross-over athlete* finds an unexpected opportunity to revive an athletic career in a totally different direction—a direction that is not fraught with the traumatic injuries often associated with the ball sports. Again, the former athlete is handed a new lease on life.

• Type 3—For the *nonathlete,* aerobic sport offers a fantasy come true. Bitter youthful memories of never making the team can be at least partially erased by taking up an aerobic sport, adopting the aerobic lifestyle, and hey, maybe in the local 10K road race, beating by more than 5 minutes the football tackle who used to be your worst nightmare in homeroom.

Aerobic sports have so much going for them that it's easy to see how grown people could become so enthralled—as enthralled as if they'd found the fountain of youth.

Unfortunately, everything under the sun has its dark side.

A CLASSIC EXAMPLE: JIM FIXX (TYPE 3)

Although he never won a road race and never competed in the Olympic Games, Jim Fixx was one of the most recognized runners in the world during the period between 1977 and 1984. His fame began with the publication in the autumn of 1977 of a book titled *The Complete Book of Running* that became a runaway best-seller, and it grew from there until nearly every advertisement having to do with running featured Fixx in some way. He also had the distinction of starring in the first video on running.

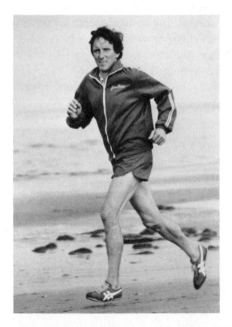

Running author Jim Fixx stuck faithfully to a regimen of 10 miles per day and stayed faithful to his belief that running had provided a much-needed anchor in his life. (Copyright J.A. Bilbao, courtesy of Random House)

Life was not always so filled with health, fame, and success for Fixx. At the age of 43, Fixx's father died of heart disease. He had suffered his first heart attack at 35.

There are many factors that, singly or in combination, predispose a person to heart disease and, ultimately, death. The more factors present, the greater the risk. Some factors in combination—for instance, cigarette smoking, high blood pressure, and obesity—tend to greatly multiply the chances of heart disease.

The risk factors range from those we can control (smoking, high blood pressure, body fat, stress, high dietary cholesterol, sedentary lifestyle) to black-on-white life statistics over which we have no control: age, sex, race, and family history.

When his father suffered his fatal heart attack at age 43, Fixx was strapped into the classic American heart disease roller coaster. He was male and was both obese and a regular smoker; he worked a series of high-stress jobs in the editorial departments of a succession of top-drawer New York City–based magazines: *Saturday Review, McCall's,* and *Life.* His diet was atrocious: extremely high in blood vessel–clotting cholesterol; his obesity and diet were contributing to high blood pressure; his father had a history of heart disease; and Jim's age was creeping up on him. Heart disease had found a crumbling house into which it could release its termites.

In 1967, at age 35 (the age at which his father experienced his first heart attack), Fixx took up running to heal a calf injury he had suffered playing tennis. Although running was difficult because of his excess weight, Fixx stuck with it and went so far as to participate in his first road race over Memorial Day weekend that year in Greenwich, Connecticut; he finished in last place, though a photo of him sporting his number 154 shows him smiling and in good spirits as he jogged along in front of the police Cushman three-wheeler bringing up the back of the pack.

By sticking with his running program, Fixx saw the pounds melt away, and he no longer finished at the back of the pack. A photo of him at the 1974 edition of the same Memorial Day race shows a slim, happy guy glorying in his hard-won health. He had not yet significantly changed his eating habits, but he had long since quit smoking.

A year later, fired from his editorial job, he made the second most momentous decision of his life: With two small brain-teaser books to his credit, he decided to abandon the crazy world of magazine editing in favor of writing books.

But what to write about?

Easy.

Since he'd begun running, he had been devouring everything he could find on the subject. And, since every writing course tells you to begin your book-writing career by picking something of particular interest to you, Fixx picked running—which was very important to him personally but which, in 1975, was a very unlikely topic for the general public.

He secured a modest advance on the book from Random House. Both author and publisher figured the book *might* sell enough copies to the slightly increasing number of people taking up running to at least break even. (They hoped for a 25,000 sale.)

What neither Fixx nor Random House realized was that the potential audience for such a book would be somewhat different 2 years hence. A great deal had changed between the time when Fixx landed the contract and the New York City Marathon in 1977 when the book, *The Complete Book of Running*, landed with a resounding *thud!* in the bookstores, rebounding from there to the top of the nation's bestseller lists, where it settled in for a long, long siege. (As of January 1989, the book had sold 977,913 hardback copies.)

The bright red cover with the sinewy leg (yes, it *was* Fixx's very own leg) on the verge of releasing all of that stored-up energy became a rallying point for what had become an explosion of runners in the United States.

Fixx wrote of running with an undisguised love and affection and a faith in its curative powers because he had, after all, been saved by running. He was talking from experience, from his own innermost recesses. He was living, breathing proof of the magic elixir. He had taken up running after years of abusing himself, and look what it had done for him! Look at that leg! That wasn't the leg of a fatty! That was the leg of a dyed-in-the-wool, real honest-to-God runner. Fixx had found the religion of temporal salvation, and that religion was endurance running.

He wrote on his subject in a clear and unwavering manner, and the hordes of new runners, who in 1977 were at the point where Fixx himself had been 10 years earlier, knew a kindred spirit when they read him. Jim Fixx, fun runner, runner for health and well-being, became a legend in his own time; he became that rarest of men: a man with viable answers to thorny questions.

His dream of taking up the writing life and becoming something of the hermit that one must be when writing for a living was forever negated by his first major project.

Between the book's publication in 1977 and the 1984 Olympic Games in Los Angeles, Fixx was the most prominent, most publicized non-world-class runner spokesman for the sport of running in the world.

He wrote a follow-up book on running and followed that one with a very unsuccessful book called *Jackpot!*, which told how his fame had come about; he followed that with *The Complete Book of Sports Performance*. For many years Random House published an annual Jim Fixx running diary. His books were translated into numerous languages. He appeared on radio and television talk shows, made the first video released on how to run, was quoted widely in newspapers, and was a spokesman for a variety of products and services, including Quaker Oats.

Although he was not a man who sought publicity, he made a genuine effort to represent himself and his sport well when he was in front of the cameras. His face on a television commercial, however, elicited snarls from some Americans just as passionate in their sedentary lifestyles as he was active in his.

He continued to run faithfully and he raced regularly, although he never managed to reach the level where he could break 3 hours in the marathon. He was literally addicted to running 10 miles a day, a level at which double digits seemed to hold the meaning of life. It was only extraordinary conditions that could keep Fixx from his appointed runs.

But at about 5:30 p.m. on July 20, 1984, along Highway 15 in Hardwick, Vermont, Fixx returned from a run. The day was extremely hot and humid, and Jim had been forced to cut the run short of his usual 10 miles. He fell to the roadside across from the Village Motel, where he was registered. He was dead of cardiac arrhythmia: another victim of coronary artery disease. He was 52 years old.

As word of the tragedy hit the news services, the first response of most runners was disbelief, and then personal grief as though they had lost a friend, a running partner. From many on the sedentary side of life, the response was one of unabashed glee; Fixx's death allowed them a momentary victory in a war of increasing defeats, to the glory of a sedentary "deathstyle."

The autopsy performed on Fixx uncovered severe closure of both the left and right coronary arteries, 97 to 99 percent on the former and 80 to 85 percent on the latter. A third coronary artery was 40 to 45 percent closed, while the remaining three arteries were partially obstructed. Arteriosclerosis had been silently at work in Fixx's arteries for decades, and although his running strengthened his heart, his past physical abuse (smoking, bad diet, stress, and so on) and his hereditary tendencies conspired to demand their inevitable toll.

In addition to the severe artery closure, it was discovered that the coronary incident that killed Fixx was not the only one he had had. It was found that the heart had been working against increasingly losing odds, possibly for months. Scar tissue, both healed and new, was found on the heart muscle, evidence that Fixx had begun having minor heart attacks months before his death, including attacks as recently as 2 weeks before the final one.

He had been urged to have stress tests over the years (most recently by Cooper during a visit Fixx made to Cooper's Aerobics Institute in Dallas), but he almost religiously—nearly pathologically—avoided them. Some felt that, quite familiar with his father's history and knowledgeable about the workings of the heart from his research on running and exercise, he did not want to face a prognosis of what was almost certainly his preordained fate. They theorized that Fixx preferred to enjoy the additional years he'd won himself by altering his lifestyle and did not want to hear a doctor's prediction of how much time he had left or, perhaps worse yet, the admonition that with the encroaching heart problem, he'd best forget running. Running was Fixx's salvation, and he was as addicted to it as a drug addict is to his or her (no pun) fix.

This is a sentiment that a sedentary person would never understand. But it is a sentiment with which a person deeply involved in endurance exercise can sympathize.

Fixx did not die from taking an endurance sport to wretched excess. In fact, all evidence points to just the opposite: that dedication to an endurance sport likely lengthened his life (although it might have been additionally lengthened had he run a bit less and had he significantly altered his diet and monitored his condition with periodic stress tests).

The real question that his death raised was whether or not he would have been willing to give up his dedication to running in order to prolong his life a bit longer still if he had to face those extra years stripped of the psychological lift running gave him.

Actually, that is the real question raised not by Fixx's death, but by his unwillingness to chance having his running removed permanently from his life.

3

CHAPTER

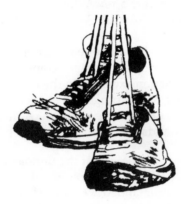

THE FIX

Instant gratification is reaching epidemic proportions in the United States and, by example, in other countries.

Whereas at one time it was accepted that if a person wanted something, acquiring it would take a certain amount of work and patience, that is not the case these days. Patience and long-term goals are becoming a thing of the past.

It is increasingly common to hear of "menial" jobs going begging while unemployed people pass those jobs by because to accept one would "demean their dignity," because "there's no future in it" or "it's not compatible with my image of myself." They prefer to accept welfare, which somehow no longer demeans one's dignity. At the same time, there are still a handful of hard-working people who take several menial jobs to support their families while striving for a better life and who don't seem to feel that their dignity has been compromised.

Life in these United States has in some ways been made too easy, and instant gratification—or at least the *expectation* of instant gratification—has become too common.

An infant begins to cry and the mother instantly picks it up, teaching the child that it can train the mother to provide instant gratification.

A teenager can't wait to get out of high school to earn a paycheck and buy material things that will satisfy the need for instant gratification. Or worse yet, the teen can't wait to drop out of high school and satisfy a need to be instantly finished with that unpleasant phase of life. It is increasingly unthinkable to invest a few additional years for potentially greater rewards farther down the road. Some high schools report 50 percent dropout rates.

Even college graduates, who have invested additional years in preparing for a profession, frequently exhibit the instant gratification syndrome, expecting to walk from graduation exercises to the top rung of a corporate ladder without hitting any of the rungs in between.

Newsweek (Myturn, 1988) detailed the problem. A mother with a fresh college graduate on her hands put it this way:

> Then one day, when she was looking at the Sunday paper and complaining that there was nothing in it, I told her there *had* to be something. 'Look at this,' I commanded. 'And this! And this!' I circled a number of jobs in the first two columns I skimmed. But Maureen protested: 'I don't want to be an administrative assistant.'

> It was then that her father and I realized that she had been looking in the paper for a career, not a job. And ever since, we have watched the children of friends suffer from this same delusion. No one, it seems, has told them that a career is an evolutionary process. (p. 52)

This attitude extends to every corner of existence. There's the weight loss instant gratification syndrome. Most people who are pathological about losing weight would never think of investing a half hour every other day in an exercise routine aimed at weight control. The rewards would be too remote in time to even be considered. These folks would rather wait for the next lose-weight-quick diet shouted from the front page of a checkout stand tabloid.

It seems never to occur to those bent on instant gratification that a pattern of frustration and disappointment awaits.

The child who was always picked up upon demand emerges into the real world and finds that the rest of the world, with wants and needs of its own, does not respond on its command as its mother did. The child ends up frustrated and bitter.

For the high school dropout, the instant gratification of escaping homework and "teacher's dirty looks" is quickly replaced by the realization that there's nothing to do and nowhere to go, that life's a dead end in a world that is increasingly complex, technologically oriented, and demanding of some educational background. And of course one wouldn't want to compromise one's dignity by working at a fast-food restaurant, or compromise one's pride by dropping back into school to complete the education.

College graduates who want to start at the top? Good luck.

And wonder diet addicts? By this time they know the yo-yo routine, but they still live in desperate hope of a quick and easy cure.

Where did this obsession with instant gratification begin?

To some extent, it's always been around, but traditionally it has belonged to the realm of the well-to-do—those who could afford to pay the tab. "Reginald is graduating from prep school this month, and he wants a new Stutz-Bearcat? But of course he shall have it!"

The startling thing about the current obsession with instant gratification is that it is not confined to those who can afford it. It has become the obsession of the masses.

And it has been fed by various segments of society.

Perhaps the first to feed it were the retail and banking communities.

In 1950, if a middle-class family wanted a television set but lacked the money to buy it, they were likely to begin saving a little each week until they had enough for the purchase. Or they might use a layaway plan, where the store put the TV away in a back room, and the family paid $5 a week until the set was paid for and it was theirs. That was pretty much the antithesis of instant gratification.

But gradually merchants began to realize that they could move more merchandise faster and avoid cluttering up their warehouses if they gave credit, either underwritten by a bank or floated on the store's books. Now a family could walk in, pick out a TV set, sit down with the store manager and negotiate a loan through either the store or the local bank, and walk out an hour later with the television.

This worked so well that merchants and banks thought up newer, better, and *faster* ways to expedite the process. Voilà! The credit card. Essentially, an instant loan. Walk into the store, pick out the television, slap that piece of plastic down on the counter, and 5 minutes later that TV's in your GMAC-financed car and on its way to the top shelf of the credit card–financed video cabinet in your bank-financed condo or house.

To save up the money and to go into a store and pay cash for a major item these days is to take a chance on baffling the salesperson or perhaps inducing a stroke or heart attack. Try it some time. Faced with the threat of someone paying for a television with cash, the salesperson is confused, disoriented, sometimes even resentful.

What does this long discussion of instant gratification have to do with exercise addiction? Patience, please. No instant gratification here.

A Self-Test
Measure Your Patience Quotient

On a scale of 1 to 10, with 10 being the strongest response, give an objective weight to each of the following statements as they apply to you and your patience in daily life. Then total your numbers and see the computations at the end of this test.

_____ I enjoy films where the problem is resolved by the time the film is over; films that leave the ending unresolved leave me flat.

_____ One of the world's biggest wastes of time is standing in line—any line.

_____ In aerobic training, short-term goals are much more important—and satisfying—than long-term goals.

_____ Stephen King horror novels are much too long and drawn out and take too long to read.

_____ A camcorder has it all over a 35mm camera.

_____ In school, I much preferred taking a test for a class grade to doing a term paper.

_____ I tend to send my federal income tax forms in right at the April 15 deadline and occasionally need an extension.

_____ When I've got a plane to catch, I regularly make it to the gate barely in time.

_____ There are too few hours in the day.

_____ I prefer dropping exposed photographic film off at 1-hour drive-up services rather than taking it to the drugstore.

_____ I drive in the fast lane on multilane highways even when I'm not passing anyone.

_____ As a spectator sport, football is better than baseball.

_____ Automatic bank teller machines are one of the greatest inventions of this decade.

_____ Most of the daily business I conduct is done over the phone; the mail is far too slow.

_____ He who hesitates is lost.

_____ TOTAL

Where does your total fall? 131-150, instant gratification specialist; 101-130, leanings toward instant gratification; 71-100, average impatience; 41-70, mild impatience; 10-40, generally patient.

I'd invested quite a bit of time over the last decade contemplating aerobic exercise addiction and how it works. But my thought process never took such a quantum leap as it did following a November 13, 1987, interview with Brooks Johnson, director of track and cross-country at Stanford University in Palo Alto, California.

I had known Johnson for several years because of my association with *Runner's World*. The magazine for many years sponsored a series of track races between American corporations known as The Corporate Cup. For most of its years, the event was held at the Stanford University track, and Johnson served as liaison between Stanford and *Runner's World*, not always an easy job. He is a very good coach and, like good coaches around the world, has his own unique theories. They apparently work, because in a school noted for its academics, he's managed to coach quite a few athletes to outstanding performances and national honors. In recognition of his achievements, Johnson served as women's track and field coach of the U.S. Olympic Team in 1984.

I had gone by Stanford to talk with him about how to safely bring student athletes out of the off-season and into top form by the time track and field started in the spring. I was doing a piece for *Sports Care & Fitness* and was interviewing a number of high school and college track coaches.

During the interview he went off on a tangent, as frequently happens in conversation with him. The tangent had to do with the predominance of black Americans in sprint events and their scarcity in distance events,

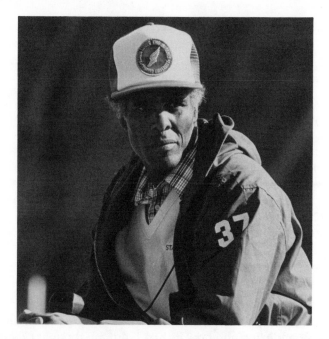

Brooks Johnson is the director of track and cross country at Stanford University in Palo Alto, California. He served as women's track coach for the 1984 US Olympic Team. He has some very unique ideas about instant and delayed gratification. (Courtesy of Stanford University/Davis Photography)

especially the marathon. Mentioning the marathon in Johnson's presence is certain to create an entire roadmap of tangents.

He pointed out that the tendency of black Americans to dominate the sprint events was of fairly recent vintage. He mentioned that in the 1970s one of the biggest names in sprint events was the Russian Valery Borzov (gold medal in the 100 and 200 meters in the 1972 Olympics, bronze medal in the 100 meters in the 1976 Olympics).

His theory as to why black Americans these days gravitate to the sprints and white Americans to the distance events involved instant gratification. White Americans, he contended, were frequently raised with the Protestant work ethic and taught a willingness to delay gratification, while to survive in modern society, black Americans were raised on instant gratification. Consequently, black Americans did not perform well in college—because both college itself and the procedures for testing and grading in college are based upon delayed gratification. (Consider the term paper, a long-term project in which gratification—a grade—comes a long time after the work is begun.)

Black Americans, Johnson held, could see the results of their efforts in sprint races almost instantly, and in the track world significant monetary rewards traditionally went along with doing well in that arena. Marathon running, on the other hand, had only recently begun to offer enough money to be worthwhile; moreover, it promised no instant gratification. There were some stark contrasts between the two sports:

1. A marathoner, because of the preparation necessary, could perform well only two or three times a year, while a sprinter could race well several times a week.

2. Gratification from sprinting came as little as 10.5 seconds after the starting gun; in the marathon, gratification typically came more than 2 hours after the start.

3. The training psychology was totally different: The sprinter went to the track, did the warm-up, did the practice, cooled down, and went home; a marathon runner's workout might last for hours and be very boring.

Although Johnson's observations held some water in their application to the sprints and the marathon, I didn't agree with the wider social theories his observations implied. I knew too many white Americans who had spent their entire lives dedicated to instant gratification and who still ended up doing marathons, and I had known certain black Americans who were excellent students (and who functioned very well in the academic world of delayed gratification) despite having numerous siblings who did not.

During the next week or two, however, my discussion with Johnson kept coming back to mind. And his observations on instant gratification—*minus* the racial implications—began making more and more sense in the context of exercise in general and exercise addiction in particular.

One of the great failings associated with regular exercise in our society is the incredibly high dropout rate. James M. Rippe (Oldridge, 1982), assistant professor of medicine and director of the exercise physiology laboratory in the Division of Cardiovascular Medicine, University of Massachusetts Medical Center, Worcester, cited studies showing more than a 50 percent dropout rate among exercisers during the first 6 months to a year. The dropout rate, I contend, is the fault not of the exercise, but of the psychology that the exerciser brings to the regimen. Too many people see the results of exercise in others, want the same results in themselves, take up exercise, and become bored or discouraged when they are not instantly gratified to find themselves metamorphosed overnight into Greek gods or goddesses.

Conversely, psychology explains why successful business executives were able to stick with Cooper's program of 20 minutes a day 3 or 4 days a week when the exercise never lasted long enough to become enjoyable in itself. These executives stuck with the program, some for 20 years, because they were used to long-term goals and delayed gratification. One does not become successful in business through an obsession with instant gratification. A good business executive needs the ability to set short- and long-term goals and to plan carefully for results that may not bear fruit for several years, sometimes even for decades.

A fitness program based upon exercise does not mesh with an appetite for instant gratification. Results in such a program come to the person who is willing to work hard at delaying the gratification. To a point.

THE PURITAN WORK ETHIC REWARDED

As easy as it is to be critical of the single-minded work ethic that was passed down to much of America through examples set by the early settlers, the philosophy that "you get what you work for" can be easily defended.

Much of the criticism of the Puritan work ethic that dominated America's early settlements focuses on the dour outlook of those Puritans. They were seemingly so taken with hard work as a purifying medium that they seldom took time to enjoy the results.

The philosophy that hard work produces lasting results was not lost on the myriad immigrants who made up the unique mixture of races, religions, and ethnic backgrounds that constituted America a century ago. Polish Catholics were as likely to respond to the Puritan work ethic as were a colony of Quakers.

Because of the forms of governments prevailing in many of the countries that produced America's early settlers, hard work was not always rewarded—the fruit of that work frequently went into the hands of the ruling class, and the hard-working peasant was left with little.

In America, with its cornucopia of opportunities and its wealth of natural resources, people willing to work hard were likely to reap more of the profits for themselves than in their native countries. Those with a spark of imagination and inventiveness might be able to start businesses of their own and enjoy even more of the fruits of their labor.

The fact that one could work hard and succeed in America is what continues to draw immigrants, many of whom apply themselves with enthusiasm and high hopes and end up reaping the fabled benefits.

In considering endurance activities, the Puritan work ethic applies. No matter how much genetic talent one brings to an endurance sport, doing well requires the investment of substantial time and effort. Aerobic sports do not lend themselves to loafing or to fabricating workouts. While a genetically endowed athlete might be able to muscle his way through a 100-meter sprint, no marathoner has ever won a race without putting in a great deal of work.

As outlined in chapter 2, the hard work invested in an aerobic sport is suitably rewarded in a variety of physical and psychological ways: with better cardiovascular health, increased self-esteem, lower blood pressure, tension relief, increased muscle tone and strength, and so forth.

While fast-paced sports and sports that require rather violent explosions of energy favor the genetically endowed (and this is not to say that football players, basketball players, sprinters, and the like do not have to work at their sports), endurance sports are more democratic. In an endurance sport, a less genetically endowed individual who trains harder and smarter is likely to be able to beat a more genetically endowed individual who does not train as hard.

Although he is certainly genetically endowed, marathoner Bill Rodgers used to train faithfully and well. He gloried in training on particularly miserable days (hot and muggy, rainy and windy) because his philosophy was this: "I know that while I'm out here training my ass off today in this miserable weather, at least some of the guys who are going to line up against me next Sunday are still home in bed." It must have worked, because besides twice holding the American marathon record, Rodgers enjoyed a period in 1978 when he won 22 road races in a row, at every distance from the 10K to the marathon.

Another perfect example of hard work yielding discernible results in endurance events is Emil Zatopek, the legendary Czech distance runner. Zatopek trained at a capacity that would have killed or crippled a lesser man, and that ultimately did cripple him temporarily. Even while he was in the Czech army, he would train while on guard duty by running in place or by running back and forth in his full uniform and military boots along the sector of fence he was guarding. Zatopek remains the only person ever to have won all three distance events (5,000 meters, 10,000 meters, and marathon) in one Olympic Games (1952).

In endurance training, one's progress is easily measured by very perceivable results. A person who begins a modest jogging program and struggles through a mile in 12:37 during the first day will quickly see improvement as hard work is applied and the program moves forward. In 6 weeks the typical mile time may be down to 10:47; in 12 weeks, the mile may fall to under 10 minutes. The benefits of weight loss, additional energy in the leg muscles, and growing self-esteem become obvious.

The exerciser who takes up an endurance training program and sticks with it, then, is guaranteed ongoing positive feedback from the body and from the mind, and quite likely from friends and family who note the changes and applaud the accomplishments. The changes do not come overnight, certainly, but if the budding aerobic athlete is willing to forego instant gratification and take the longer view, it quickly becomes apparent that hard work equals rewards.

The trick in aerobic sports, of course, is to know just how much hard work is good, and where to draw the line at doing so much hard work that it becomes counterproductive.

Rest days and easy days are as important as hard-work days in making an aerobic program successful. Brooks Johnson, the Stanford coach I cited in the last section, is a firm believer that of the four basic elements of training, rest is the most important element, and frequently the one that is ignored.

But the fact remains that hard work eventually brings results—and usually rewards. Still, while hard work is rewarded in aerobic sports (in a confirmation of the Puritan work ethic), it is easy for an overly enthusiastic exerciser to end up doing too much, to his or her own undoing.

Just as the workaholic becomes obsessed with the job to avoid dealing with troubles at home, and just as the workaholic is often the least productive person at the office because she or he is obsessed with the idea of work rather than with the smooth and effective execution of that work, so, too, the aerobic exerciser is capable of going overboard in physical activity, of using it to put off dealing with personal problems, and ultimately of abusing it.

The aerobic arena is also quite capable of providing a great deal of pain and discomfort to the person inclined to such abuse.

THE MARTYR SYNDROME

Some people seem to find fulfillment in suffering—and they aren't necessarily raving masochists. To some of these people, in suffering there is moral nobility.

Many people who suffer stoically and many who suffer pain grandly are taught to do so from a very young age. Many religions teach that it is noble to suffer and that to enjoy life on this earth is in some way sinful. A child taught this philosophy is essentially prepared to accept pain and suffering throughout life, not only as a way of life but as a route to salvation. As, if you will, a desirable thing.

An example of this philosophy taken to the extreme can be found in east-central Pennsylvania in the town of Ephrata. The commonwealth of Pennsylvania maintains a historic site called the Ephrata Cloisters. It is the site of a short-lived religious group that came from Germany; they believed that one's position in the afterlife was directly proportional to the suffering endured in this life. Consequently, the designers of the cloisters took every opportunity to offer discomfort: Members slept in small, unheated cells on bare-board beds with brick-shaped wooden pillows; they ate the most meager of foods; they slept no more than 2 hours at a time; and they were awakened at midnight for church services. One of the sufferings they were taught to endure was segregation of male and female members. There was no social—much less sexual—intercourse between them. This, of course, proved to be the cult's undoing: With no social structure to encourage courting and marriage (and consequently children), the cult died out. Obviously, an example of short-term planning.

Virtually every Christian sect, while not as fanatical as the cult that lived in Ephrata, is based upon the concept of reward for suffering. The ultimate sufferer and reward recipient, of course, is the martyr: that person who makes the ultimate sacrifice—of one's life—for religion.

Sports and exercise (both aerobic and anaerobic) are saturated with this same philosophy of gain from pain. It goes under the oft-shouted and oft-inscribed motto of "No pain, no gain!"

This philosophy is rife among football players and bodybuilders. Football and bodybuilding workouts lend themselves to quick, explosive efforts that sear the nerves in muscles, that cause a burning sensation, and that can be considered painful.

The pain in endurance sports training (unless an injury is involved) is typically an all-encompassing discomfort that can last for a very long time. Endurance sports, then, are more compatible with religious endurance of suffering because they provide opportunities for extended suffering. Just as a novice in the Ephrata Cloisters was uncomfortable for 2 hours trying to sleep on a board, and as a religious layperson might be uncomfortable during an hour of kneeling on a hard board in a pew, so a 4-hour marathoner may be extremely uncomfortable for the last 90 minutes of a marathon.

Suffering in endurance sports is offered on two fronts:

1. The *amorphous physical discomfort* of training or racing as the body tires and ultimately exhausts itself, often to the point of "hitting the wall" in running or "bonking" in bicycling.
2. The *acute physical pain* of training or racing through an injury.

Those who are already injured and who insist on training or racing anyway have the potential to enjoy both types of suffering at once.

Joe Oakes, one of the triathlon pioneers, had just such an opportunity, you'll recall: "I was so badly into my training and competing, that 8 days after breaking three ribs, a shoulder, and my wrist [he was hit by a car while training on his bicycle], I went and did the Ironman anyway. I did the swim with my left arm, and the bike and run weren't quite so difficult. There was pain associated with it, but that's what aspirin are for."

In another instance, a group of runners competing in the 10K road race that was part of the Corporate Cup at Berkeley a decade ago were horrified to see a competitor running along striking himself on the buttocks and hamstrings with a switch he'd torn off a tree. I don't know if the self-abuse spurred the flagellant on, but it certainly spurred my frends and me to double our efforts to get away from the weirdo.

The consideration of a martyr syndrome involving pain and suffering in endurance sports is not meant to imply that everyone who engages in such a sport is into it for its masochistic potential. Any great physical effort carries with it the potential for pain or discomfort. Professional athletes who have trained and competed for decades accept the discomfort as a part of the package. Many of them have learned to accept acute discomfort in an almost academic manner, intellectualizing it. This is especially true of distance runners who twice a week go to the track to do repeat quarters. There is nothing serene about doing 20 quarters at 68 seconds with a half-lap jog between, yet most accomplished distance runners do the repeats because they know they need them to improve their speed.

Some aerobic athletes, however, seem to wallow in the discomfort associated with hard and long workouts or races and seem to obtain a catharsis from such experiences. It is not unusual after a hard workout is over to hear the expression, "That hurt good."

There is also the situation—very much associated with the religious teaching that suffering on this earth is good—in which a person who suffers pain and discomfort believes that he or she rises above other people, presumably in holiness and spiritual purity.

This belief has some dark comedy overtones because it seems to permeate many aspects of one-upmanship.

Several years ago, while visiting a California historical area, my wife and I began talking with two elderly people who were manning the gift shop. Somehow, after a few minutes, the conversation was swung around to coronary bypass operations (perhaps the couple was adept at this maneuver), and we were informed that both husband and wife had had multiple bypass surgery. Another elderly couple in the shop overheard this and moved over to the counter to inform all of us that they, too, had had multiple bypass surgery. At that point, the four of them began adding up how many arteries had been involved. Not to be outdone, the man behind the counter announced that he had had the operation twice!

There was never even the hint that a person who had not had bypass surgery might be better off than any one of them. Instead, the entire conversation was a duel of one-upmanship deeply mired in the martyr syndrome: I've suffered more than you have, therefore I am a better person than you are, and my chair in heaven will be higher.

Often, listening to a distance runner's description of a weekend race is not unlike hearing a religious convert enunciating his or her sufferings for the betterment of the everlasting soul:

"The conditions were atrocious."

"The heat was unreal."

"The course was horrible."

"I could hardly walk for an hour afterwards."

"My quads were in agony from the halfway point on."

"After a few hours, it got so bad that even my hair hurt."

Well, why didn't you stop when it got so bad?

"Stop? Are you crazy?"

If the intrinsic pain and suffering of an aerobic sport pushed too far can provide uplifting and fulfilling pain, there is another form of pain that is intimately involved with endurance sports that demand regularity for results: guilt. Good old American guilt.

GUILT AND THE MISSED WORKOUT

America is a nation driven by guilt.

The same Puritans who gave us the work ethic also railed against enjoying the fruits of that work.

The Puritan propensity toward restraint through guilt was augmented by Jewish and Catholic immigrants, two groups of people who have traditionally raised guilt to an art form. (In one of his films, Woody Allen makes the statement that he can't get through a day without at least one juicy rationalization. For Jews and Catholics, a day without guilt is a day one should feel guilty for living.)

I can vividly recall a time in the early 1950s when my father was out of work for an extended period. Despite our family's dire circumstances, our mother reminded us at meals of how much we had to be thankful for, and how much more we had than the poor people in China, and how we should appreciate it.

Something of a national guilt regarding the prosperity of the United States overlooks the fact that millions of people worked long and hard and were uniquely inventive in fashioning the country into what it is.

In the course of history, nations victorious in war traditionally pillage the defeated countries and turn them into colonies. Following the Second World War the United States not only helped repair the damage to its allies but also helped rebuild the economies of its enemies, Germany and Japan, to the point that 40 years later they are economic rivals. Yet Americans are made to feel guilty by the rest of the world amidst accusations of imperialism, while in reality their country bears the burden of an empire (footing most of the bills for the NATO alliance, for example) without enjoying any of the advantages.

The examples of national and individual guilt under which Americans labor could fill a book. The point is that guilt, in one form or another, is ever present, especially among the demographic groups that contribute the majority of endurance athletes.

Is it difficult to imagine the psychological wrestling that goes on, then, when a person becomes committed to an endurance program, makes it a regular part of life, and then faces the possibility of missing a scheduled workout? The mere contemplation of a missed workout sets off the guilt sirens, and it becomes easier just to go ahead with the workout as planned than to miss it and take on an additional guilt burden. The studious avoidance of additional guilt from missing scheduled workouts serves as one more factor in addicting the exerciser—even if the contemplated exercise is contraindicated.

- Delayed gratification
- A strict adherance to the Puritan work ethic
- The martyr syndrome
- Guilt

Each factor alone has the potential to lock a person into the addiction phase of exercise, but two or more of them combined make the addiction even more potent and difficult to break, typically fueling an ever-ascending spiral of involvement.

We feel exhilarated at our ability to postpone gratification until *after* the long workout. We feel that the hard work we are putting into the exercise is worthwhile—as the physical and psychological benefits inherent in an endurance exercise regimen would indicate. We are occasionally uplifted by our ability to suffer more physical pain and discomfort than our sedentary friends—often more than many of our macho friends in traditional sports. And we feel satisfied that we have not missed a workout in the past month and therefore have nothing to feel guilty about.

With two or more of these factors blending as the motivating force behind our workouts, and with those factors working to further addict us, the cycle becomes more difficult to break:

- Who would want to remove the short- and long-term goals that ultimately bring gratification?
- Who would want to forego the physical and psychological benefits?
- Who would want to undermine our principles of ultimately receiving what we work for?
- Who would want to give up the suffering that sets us apart from the rest of mankind?

To remove the endurance sport would be to bring down the ravages of guilt—ravages that we could not very well withstand because they involve guilt from undermining good works we've undertaken to improve ourselves.

And the very existence of those good works done on our own behalf for our own betterment merely adds one more factor to an already complex blend of motivations to keep going, no matter what the cost.

THE ADDICTION TO REWARD

Another very significant ingredient should be added to the stewpot of factors promoting addiction to endurance sport, and that is the ingredient of plain, unadulterated reward.

Employees of major corporations who are unhappy with their jobs frequently cite as their major complaint the fact that they are not appreciated, that they are not complimented on their work, that they are not rewarded or recognized enough.

Imagine the limited expectations of the nonathlete who takes up an endurance sport. Here is a person who, as a youngster, received no positive feedback when participating in sport and may have actually endured verbal abuse ("Ah, ya can't even see the ball, much less hit it!"). Here is a person who, through adulthood, accepted being effectively barred from sports for a lack of certain talents typically associated with those sports. Now, later in life, this same person finds that aerobic sports are readily accessible and reward perseverance and dedication with a raft of benefits.

But the complication goes well beyond that. Besides the physical and psychological benefits outlined previously, there are very real rewards for those who compete in races.

The typical century bicycle race awards commemorative patches to all finishers. Running races give commemorative T-shirts, as do swimming events. Citizen cross-country ski races award patches and pins. Triathlons give T-shirts, caps, swim caps, and a bag of goodies. Some major marathons give medals to all finishers.

In addition to these symbolic awards, the participants receive tremendous tactical support from volunteer groups manning aid stations and get emotional and spiritual support from spectators. The names of the finishers are printed in race result booklets sent to all competitors, and the newspapers in some cities print the names of all who finish. And for racers who are reasonably competitive, there are age-group awards, given more and more frequently to a depth that reflects the percentage of total participants coming from a particular age group.

Another very positive factor is associated with competition: support and admiration from family, friends, and coworkers.

Many aerobic athletes who become involved in competition are at first overwhelmed by the attention and special treatment they receive. This is especially true for those who have never been athletes before. The attention, the notoriety come as a shock—a very pleasant shock.

Rapidly, the competitor begins to expect this type of positive feedback at races, this coddling that is perhaps not present in any other aspect of life. And little by little, the competitor not only expects it but begins to thrive on it, until it seems inconceivable that he or she had ever lived without the attention, the genuine concern, the finite rewards. (Even the most accomplished local hotshot runner is not immune to this expectation. A friend of mine who is a top distance runner in the Bay Area proudly hangs all of his hundreds of race T-shirts in a special closet, where they are arranged by colors, creating a rainbow effect for the unwary visitor who naively opens the wrong closet door.)

It is very easy, then, to become addicted to the positive feedback received during a race, to the symbolic rewards like T-shirts and medals, and to the support and admiration of family and friends.

Considering all the potentially addicting ingredients of an aerobic lifestyle, it is no wonder that addiction is common among the aerobically fit.

HOW COMMON IS ADDICTION?

With the potentially addicting allures of an endurance lifestyle as a background, this would seem a convenient spot—before looking at other factors that cement the addiction—to ask just how many aerobic athletes are actually addicted.

As with other discussions of aerobic athletes, most studies have focused on the long-distance runner. This is primarily due to the large numbers of subjects available following the running revolution of the late 1970s, to the ease of pinpointing the more serious runners by their participation in one or more of the thousands of road races held annually around the country, and to the tendency of these people to respond to questionnaires and other research efforts. The results of studies involving runners can typically be extended to other aerobic athletes in most respects. A notable exception is activity-related injuries: Each activity—because of the specific muscles used and risks involved—tends to occasion certain injuries.

Before considering research that puts percentages to addiction in running, we should briefly consider the distinct possibility that *commitment* and *addiction* are not necessarily the same.

You'll recall that, in chapter 1, we cited research by Carmack & Martens (1979) on commitment to running. They surveyed 315 runners (250 male, 65 female), using a five-page questionnaire that took 20 to 30 minutes to complete. The questionnaire was divided into five parts:

1. Demographic information of a general nature
2. Questions specific to running
3. Questions regarding state of mind during the run (22 items)
4. Commitment to running scale (12 items)
5. Perceived outcomes of running (40 items)

The survey was effective and thorough, although it served to confirm already held observations about commitment rather than to apprehend new and startling information. The survey was so thorough that it in effect became a standard test to measure runner commitment.

Dale Pierre Layman (1986) used the Carmack and Martens commitment test as a portion of a much more ambitious research project that served as his PhD dissertation, "The Runner: A Profile of Injury and Addiction." Layman attempted to uncover correlations between a runner's addiction to running and the incidence and severity of running-related injuries.

The survey that was the basis of Layman's dissertation involved 1,227 subjects. It is instructive to review the statistical profile of those subjects, both to establish a better feel for the typical long-distance runner and to further confirm preceding discussions of this group from a demographic standpoint.

Of the 1,227 subjects, 1,039 had suffered some sort of running-related injuries during their involvement—injuries serious enough to cause the subjects to cancel runs on subsequent days because of the injury's incapacitating nature.

Of the 1,039 subjects who had been injured, 62.3 percent (647) were male and 37.7 percent (392) were female. Average age was 34.70. The group as a whole had been running for an average of 75.21 months with a regularity of 4.78 days per week, averaging a distance of 30.21 miles per week. Nearly 81 percent had participated in a race or races during the previous year.

From an educational standpoint, 21.8 percent had earned a 4-year college degree, and 37.1 percent had elected some formal graduate work. More than half (52 percent) were employed in a managerial or professional capacity.

Layman divided his subjects into three general age groups: young (25 and under), middle-aged (26 to 40), and mature (above 40).*

The largest age category, not surprisingly, was 26 to 40, which accounted for 47.8 percent of the total.

The mean age of male runners was 4 years higher than the mean age of females, and the typical male had been running 14 months longer than the typical female. Of the total sample, Layman found that 63.2 percent qualified as runners and the remaining 36.8 percent as joggers.

Layman set out to determine which of the runners in his survey group were committed, objectively addicted, and subjectively addicted. Because of the quality of its past performance, he used the Carmack and Martens test of commitment. Layman stated:

---

*Most endurance athletes who participate in their sport at least in part to hold off the aging process would likely take exception to Layman's defining 26 to 40 as middle-aged; they are still attempting to fight off the traditional stereotype of 40 to 59 as being middle-aged!

Since a major focus of this research was on addiction to running, an important question concerned the identity or relatedness of the three purported measures of addiction to running utilized in the study: subjective addiction to running, objective addiction to running, and commitment to running. Although review of the literature had pointed out that Commitment to Running has often been viewed as synonymous with addiction to running, it was the belief of the researcher that addiction to running involved something above and beyond mere commitment to the physical activity. Statistical evidence to support this supposition came from correlational analysis, cross-tabulation, and factor analysis. (p. 135)

Following an explanation of each of these analyses, Layman concluded "that commitment to running is a closely related, but not identical, measure [to addiction]."

When Layman further studied his material, he found, as one would expect, that the number of runners (67.2 percent) who tested as addicted was significantly larger than the number of joggers (35.2 percent) who were addicted. A surprising statistic emerged as he checked addiction by gender. While 51.4 percent of all males tested as addicted, a startling 61.9 percent of females tested as addicted. (It is only my surmise, but this rather notable difference may be due to the fact that nearly every female runner, because of past societal restrictions, came to running as a nonathlete and was therefore more susceptible to the allures of the sport than were the males, many of whom had already been sport participants, especially in high school or college.)

Layman's statistical observation that commitment to running is not necessarily synonymous with addiction to running is consistent with my personal observations of long-distance runners over more than a decade. His findings in the percentages of joggers and runners who are addicted to their sport also mesh with my observations.

In an article titled "Addicted to Exercise," Connie Chan, clinical psychologist and assistant professor of human services at the University of Massachusetts at Boston (1986), stated that

the 'typical' exercise addict is between ages 20 and 60, female or male, and began exercising in adulthood as a way to lose weight and become more physically fit. As these individuals improve their heart rate, lose weight, and feel better physically, they also begin to feel better about themselves. They develop a sense of control over their bodies—something they had been unable to do through dieting—and this feeling of control generalizes to a sense of control over their lives. In other words, they feel more powerful and more self-confident. (p. 430)

According to the 1987 Gallup Leisure Activities Index, nearly 20 million adult Americans jog or run regularly. If we were to halve that number to cut out those who jog once or twice a week, we'd still have 10 million people in our national study group. Layman found that 55.4 percent of his subjects were addicted. Correlating the conservative Gallup number with those findings, we would come out with 5,540,000 adult Americans (of both sexes) who are addicted to their jogging or running. This number, of course, does not take into account participants in other aerobic sports (bicycling, triathlon, cross-country skiing, endurance swimming, aerobic dance, and so forth) who are addicted.

We must look at some of the Gallup numbers with caution. For example, the 1986 Gallup Poll found that there are 70,400,000 swimmers in the United States, a number that seems patently absurd and is skewed by the fact that anyone who goes to a beach and steps into the water considers him- or herself a swimmer. Of course, few of that number are long-distance swimmers capable of doing a mile or more in a session. But the point is that, when considered as a percentage of the number of participants in various aerobic sports, the number of aerobic athletes addicted to their sport becomes astronomical.

HOW THE ADDICTION PROGRESSES

Just as a combination of negative factors contributing to heart disease (for instance, cigarette smoking, heredity, and high blood pressure) creates a dangerous condition far surpassing the sum of the three factors, a combination of the factors we have discussed as contributing to aerobic addiction tends to have implications that reach far beyond the total of the individual parts.

An aerobic athlete, as we've seen, receives a raft of physical benefits (including weight control, cardiovascular health, and lower blood pressure) and psychological benefits (self-esteem, stress relief, camaraderie), and finds a socially acceptable channel for certain learned behaviors (delayed gratification, the Puritan work ethic, a tendency to martyrdom, and guilt).

The aerobic athlete has literally done for him- or herself what it would take thousands of dollars, a personal fitness coach, a weight control specialist, and a team of psychiatrists years to accomplish.

The beauty of the aerobic lifestyle is that after the initial battle to get started by getting fit in the first place (a process that, if faithfully followed, can be completed within 45 to 60 days), maintenance is not especially difficult.

Of course, as we've also seen, once the athlete is well beyond the level Cooper recommends, a whole other set of motivations cuts in, and the athlete is typically not content to merely maintain. There is the tendency, especially among the baby boomers, to go for more, to push the limits. This process, of course, is a self-sustaining exercise. The more one accomplishes, the more one wants to do.

The addiction to aerobic exercise progresses at this point primarily because of two factors:

1. The individual combination of the various physical, psychological, and learned behavior reactions to the exercise routine
2. The sudden (though often subconscious) realization that what the athlete has found is a perfectly acceptable source of not only instant, but continuous gratification

This comes as a revelation.

For the person who has been trained to believe that one must plan well and work hard for the gratification that always seems to be one step farther down the road, and who has surmised that the only way to bypass the system is through cheating or some criminal act, receiving instant gratification day after day from something as simple and basic as aerobic exercise is intoxicating—and further addicting.

Every time an aerobic exerciser looks in a mirror and sees a person with a toned, healthy body looking back, there is instant gratification. Every new race T-shirt added to the T-shirt drawer is a form of instant gratification; every time the athlete puts on one of those T-shirts to go for a workout, there is a wash of good feelings and a certain amount of gratification.

Every time an aerobic athlete walks into work and someone comments on how fit he or she looks, there is instant gratification. Every time someone inquires about the weekend's race, there is gratification. Every time the athlete manages to steer casual conversation around to a particularly difficult or grueling workout, there is gratification.

Every time aerobic athletes realize that they are more fit now than they were at half their current age, there is instant gratification. And better still, with every realization that an athlete is in better shape than most Americans who are half his or her age, there is a tremendous inrush of instant gratification.

While other company employees dread the annual physical fitness examination and stress test, aerobic athletes lose sleep the night before in anticipating how they are going to perform on the treadmill, to show the rest of the office just what fit is.

And how about continuous gratification?

Just as sickness and pain, whether acute or barely below the level of consciousness, last 24 hours a day, so too does physical fitness. A physically fit person is fit 24 hours a day and knows it—especially if she or he is surrounded by people who are *not* fit.

And the sense of continuous gratification is heightened every time the aerobic athlete double-knots the old running shoes for the daily workout, or pulls on the aerobic dance outfit, or lowers the goggles over the eyes before diving into the pool, or pumps that last extra pound of pressure into the bicycle tires.

The aerobic athlete has found the key to nirvana, the key that unlocks the closet with the secret panel that does away with delayed gratification and allows for instant gratification, and lots of it.

Denied instant gratification from childhood, the well-educated, professional American has suddenly found an arena in which gratification and rewards are virtually instant. Better yet, it is an arena of child-like sport and play that seemingly had been lost at adulthood. And still better, all of this is socially acceptable.

It is suddenly OK to be running around the neighborhood in little more than your underwear. It is all right to spend hours riding a bicycle. It is acceptable to go off frolicking in the water for an hour. In fact, it's not only acceptable, but even the stodgy family doctor says it's good for you.

Combine this exhilaration with the deep-rooted knowledge that the more you work at something the more you get from it, and you've got an addicted athlete looking to do more, more, more.

"The more I did, the more I enjoyed it," Oakes now recalls. "I ran quarter miles to start off with, because that's as far as I could go. Then 5 miles, and then 10Ks and marathons. By nature I'm more of a sprinter. But I found I enjoyed myself *more* with the 5-milers than with the sprints, and I'd go out and run them hard. Later I enjoyed running the marathons much the same way. Then the ultramarathons. Each thing that I did gave me a bit of a taste of something more than I'd done before. I guess 'more' is the word. You look at what you've done, and you say, 'Hey, I've done that. What's next? What other accomplishment is there?' "

Each accomplishment, each infusion of instant gratification calls for more. Like a sponge that has been dry for decades, these new athletes want to absorb more and more, to soak it all up.

Once they're involved, everything is going their way, at least physically, and it feels so good. The contributing factors discussed in this chapter have combined in interesting and unique ways for each individual who took up an aerobic sport, for whatever reasons, and suddenly was hooked, addicted. And these people were not above making that statement:

"I'm addicted to my running!"
"I'm hooked on aerobic dance for the rest of my life!"
"I couldn't live without my daily fix of exercise!"

These addictions developed from individual mixes of various factors, but the mixes were further cemented by the drug pusher who's above the law—one's own body.

4
CHAPTER

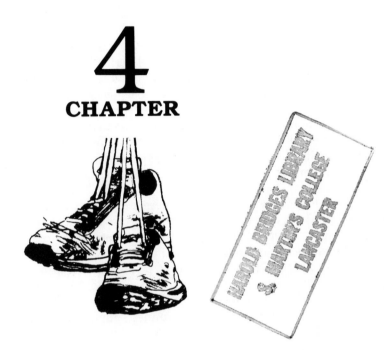

THE NATURAL
DRUG CONNECTION

Among the many passionate discussions surrounding running (jogger vs. runner, effect on bones and knees, and so on), one of the longest running involves what has been described as the *runner's high*, a feeling of power, dissociation from the body, and lightening of the physical being that infuses occasional or frequent runs, depending on the runner.

The runner's high is an almost trancelike state achieved during a run: a state of mind where the brain (or the runner's consciousness) is happy and content and seems to float above the running body, while the body seems to perform effortlessly, like a well-oiled machine or even a perpetual motion machine. The runner is elevated by the experience and during the period of "high" enjoys a pure equanimity: Problems are left behind and disturbances along the running course are overlooked or softened, while the color of the sky is heightened, the occasional bird or flower is seen as though for the first time, and the mind is emptied of its concerns, the resulting vacuum filled with the experiences of the ideal run.

In *Positive Addiction*, Glasser (1976) referred to this condition as the *positive addiction state*. One runner described the state to Glasser this way: "Your mind is there but it is not there—it's in sort of a transcendental, trancelike state." Glasser stated that "since that time I have talked to many more physically addicted people, runners and others, and it is this state of mind that almost all of them describe, a trancelike, transcendental mental state that accompanies the addictive exercise (p. 47)."

Sit down with a group of amateur runners and almost every one of them will be able to describe the feelings and experiences of the runner's high.

Not every runner experiences a high on every run. Some experience the high only occasionally, others experience it often. Some runners seem able to place themselves in such a state of mind at the beginning of a run that they create a mental environment that increases the likelihood of a high. Others who tend to be tense going into a run may need ideal circumstances for the high to occur; while they seem unable to anticipate when it will come, they tend to agree that it cannot be forced—that, in fact, attempting to force a runner's high is guaranteed to prevent it.

Runner's high does not come to the novice. There are at least five prerequisites.

1. For the uninitiated, the run must proceed through the warm-up stages so that the body becomes loose and the running begins to seem natural and smooth. This usually requires anywhere from 20 to 40 minutes of running, depending on the person and on the person's level of fitness. Some runners reportedly can induce the runner's high very early in a run; this seems to be a matter of mental training that overrides the physical awkwardness of the early minutes of running until the muscles and the breathing smooth out.

2. The runner must be sufficiently trained (in terms of conditioning) to run well beyond the warm-up period. That is, if a 1-hour run is planned, the runner must be trained well enough to be able to run comfortably beyond an hour. The runner's high does not occur when the runner is struggling to breathe properly because the run is moving into new ground physically.

3. The runner must not resist the high.

4. Experiencing the high usually requires training solo. The high is rarely reported during runs with others. And it is rarely reported in the midst of competition.

5. Perhaps most important, the running must be noncritical. This means that the runner must be running that particular run merely to be running it. The high does not come to those who are running with a critical eye toward the performance; this fact contributes to the cynicism with which national- and world-class runners regard the very concept of a runner's high. The high does not come if the runner is spending the entire run observing the performance and judging it.

Glasser (1976) made this point in *Positive Addiction*, explaining that the experience of the high is denied those who are too self-critical (such as professional athletes). "Not only must we not compete with others, we must learn not to compete with ourselves if we wish to reach the PA [positive addiction] state. That means even as we try to improve we must be careful not to criticize ourselves in the process" (p. 57).

Although this state of mind is known as the runner's high, it is experienced to some degree in virtually every aerobic sport. Because the high was first reported by and described by runners, it bears the name *runner's high* no matter what sport is involved. On the July 12, 1988, broadcast of "Running and Racing" on ESPN, Harald Johnson, former editorial director of *Triathlete* magazine, mentioned the runner's high in conjunction with his enjoyment of mountain biking in California. Consequently, the term *runner's high* is used throughout this discussion to mean *aerobic athlete's high*. Take a minute now to try the self-test, next page.

Even an athlete who is injured but is still in good physical condition and is able to participate in the sport can experience the high once the exercise has progressed to the point where the pain of the injury has been alleviated by the massaging action of the warming muscles and the body's introduction of the pain-killing opiates, the endorphins (more about them later).

The concept of the runner's high is nothing new. There are numerous examples of an altered state of consciousness in religious ceremonies throughout history, and throughout the world. The common factor among them seems to be the presence of repetitive physical activity.

Patrick J. Bird (1987), in an article titled "Runner's High Revisited," wrote:

Studies by anthropologists and psychologists have long associated strenuous physical effort with feelings of euphoria and even altered states of consciousness. One study by Wolfgang Jilek, professor of psychiatry at the University of British Columbia, for example,

A Self-Test
How "High" Do You Get
During Aerobic Sports?

There are 10 questions below. Read them carefully. For each question that elicits a Yes response, place an X on the line to the left. If your response is No, leave the line empty. When you have finished, add up the number of Xs and place that number on the line next to TOTAL.

_____ When on a workout, once you are warmed up, do you ever experience a sense of floating or flowing through some portion of that workout?

_____ In the wake of an exercise session, do you find that you cannot recall certain extended periods of the workout?

_____ Following a long workout, do you ever experience a lightheadedness and an inability to precisely coordinate motor skills (such as driving a car) for an hour or more?

_____ Are there portions of workouts that seem effortless and during which you seem to be elevated above your body?

_____ Do you sometimes seem to go on automatic pilot in the middle of a workout?

_____ Do nagging aches and pains vanish or become lessened after the first half hour of exercise?

_____ Do you occasionally experience a suspension of the sense of time midway through your exercise session?

_____ In the midst of some longer workouts, do solutions to pressing problems become clear?

_____ When workouts are missed, does it cause a sense of anxiety and dread?

_____ If you were told today that you would never again be able to exercise, would the prospect cause deep depression and emotional turmoil?

_____ TOTAL

What was your total? If it was 8-10, you've obviously experienced the fabled runner's high and you harbor the potential for some of the classic withdrawal symptoms; 5-7 indicates intimate familiarity with the runner's high; 2-4 denotes a casual acquaintance with the sensation; 0-1 indicates a lack of acquaintance.

describes altered states of consciousness experienced by initiates in North American Indian dance ceremonials (*Ethos*, Winter 1982).

The Spirit Dance, performed by the Salish tribes of British Columbia and Washington, is not a dance but rather a run to exhaustion. In this ceremony, the initiates begin by running through the woods whipping their legs with cedar branches—'in order to feel light-footed, exhilarated, and tranced.' After collapsing from the run, the runners are bathed in a hot smokehouse and then 'submerged four times in an ice-cold mountain stream.' One Salish initiate described the effect this way:

'I was jumping three feet high, and I had such a thrill, a terrific feeling as if I were floating, as if I were in the air; I felt really high. I've only had such a feeling once before in my life when I was on heroin mainlining, but then I went through hell afterwards, it was terrible. But with the spirit song's power you get this feeling without the terrible aftermath.' (p. 18, 66)

The Tarahumara Indians of northern Mexico, one of the poorest and most destitute people on earth, are underfed, undereducated, and are so uncared for medically that they have one of the highest infant mortality rates in the world.*

Yet, for all their deprivation and suffering, they are among the fittest people in the world. The tribal game, in which a wooden ball is kicked back and forth between runners, frequently covers 100 miles. A male initiation rite involves running 100 miles between sunup and sundown. Perhaps inducing a trancelike state for long periods is the only way the Tarahumara can manage to look beyond their wretched existence.

Runner's high became a phrase batted around the athletic circles when the running revolution took hold in the 1970s.

As already discussed, Glasser associated the high with his theory of positive addiction. This altered state induced by long-distance running or by meditation helped get the participant hooked on the positive addiction and helped the participant stay hooked.

Kostrubala (1976) described the experience in *The Joy of Running*.

There are certain characteristics of this phenomenon. You will know it by the quality of its appearance. I've never found it in anyone except after 40 minutes of this kind of running. It isn't always a 'peak' experience. One time it was the beauty of the red color of a fireplug.

---

*It does not help the situation that a pregnant woman who has come to term is required, by tradition, to go alone into the wilderness, find a tree with a branch just beyond her reach; and, when the time of birth comes, jump to reach the branch and cling to it until the infant is deposited on the ground below.

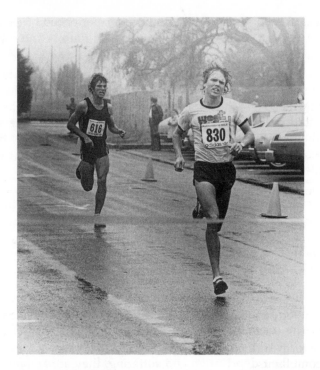

Highly competitive individuals engaged in aerobic sports seldom experience "runner's high" due to the self-critical nature of their training and competition. Dr. William Glasser's findings in the mid-1970s explained why most highly competitive runners scoffed at the concept of "runner's high." (Kenneth Lee photograph)

Just the red color, that red color, nothing more. But that red color, that time, was the nicest, neatest, brightest, finest red in the world. I could almost taste it. It happens suddenly. It's as if a trapdoor had sprung open into some secret treasure trove hiding within us. (pp. 98-99)

Earlier in the discussion he described a patient who was a "secret runner"—he ran early in the morning and kept the fact hidden lest by sharing the knowledge, he would diminish the experience.

My secret runner also described his sense of well-being and feeling refreshed after a run. He also talked about that feeling of being able to run as if he were a little off the ground—about a foot or so—and a sense of brightness and light that came near the end of his 45- to 60-minute run. (p. 94)

This feeling is the essence of the runner's high, a very pleasant, desirable experience that an athlete would like to repeat—frequently. Before exploring the biological and chemical explanations of the conditions that promote this high, let us examine the trail that scientists followed to isolate the high that feeds the running addiction, and to explain it.

A SHORT HISTORY OF HOW SCIENTISTS TRACKED DOWN A HIGH

Everyone enjoys feeling good. It is the enjoyment of feeling good that lures people into negative addictions such as drugs: For a time, use of the drug—whether cocaine, alcohol, or heroin—banishes negative feelings and elevates the addict's perceptions of the surrounding world. An overwhelming desire to travel frequently to that world of feeling good is what hooks the addict and feeds the habit.

The good feelings associated with the high of a successful aerobic workout contribute significantly to the addictive qualities of the activity. The fact that good things—physical and psychological benefits—came to those who regularly took part in aerobic activities did not escape the eye of a few psychology professionals. As a result of the insights of a handful of psychologists, psychiatrists, clinicians, and scientists, aerobic activity was used as a form of therapy for patients suffering from a variey of psychological complaints.

The early use of exercise as therapy whetted the appetites of these pioneers to learn more about the mechanisms that caused the exercise to become addictive. A brief review of the history of exericise therapy will shed more light on the phenomenon of the runner's high.

Physical activity as therapy has been known for some time, although its use was very spotty at best until the 1970s. In a major piece on the subject in *Runner's World*, Hal Higdon (1978) cited the insights of Karl Menninger, founder of the Menninger Clinic in Topeka, Kansas. "He recognized that exercise might benefit his patients, that they should be given activities such as bowling, baseball, golf, and even dancing to occupy their minds" (p. 39). At a 1977 conference on physical fitness and mental health held at the University of Nebraska, Edward Greenwood of the Menninger Foundation put it this way:

> The body and mind do not operate on different levels independent of each other. When one breaks down, the other suffers. Every change in the physiological state is accompanied by a change in the mental state; and every change in the mental state is accompanied by a change in the physiological state (p. 39).

Unfortunately, as the Menninger Clinic grew, it eventually moved away from its original attention to physical activity as a means of helping patients.

Carlyle H. Folkins, of the University of California at Davis, felt that the reason for such movement away from physical activity as therapy was one of convenience. He cited the use in the 1940s of running as a means of calming patients in the veterans' hospitals. "We went backwards," he said. "Along came tranquilizers and other forms of drugs. All the psychiatrists got out their chemistry sets and forgot about the potential benefits of exercise. It was like the old DuPont slogan: 'Better Things Through Chemistry' " (Higdon, 1978, p. 39).

It took until the 1970s for a small group of doctors—often athletic themselves—to again take up the challenge of incorporating running as therapy.

As a handful of medical folks began following clues that led them to the conclusion that physical activity had positive effects upon psychological *and* physical problems, theories were put forth to explain the mechanisms.

Psychiatrists and psychologists who used exercise—especially aerobic exercise—in their practices began to theorize that physical activity *might* burn up energy that otherwise might go into producing anxiety.

Wes Sime, director of the stress and fitness research lab at the University of Nebraska/Lincoln, held similar theories. He felt that exercise tended to reduce muscle tension and anxiety, much as meditative relaxation techniques did, and that both activities might be linked to "the total diversion from anxious cognitions."

Others, such as Pike C. Nelson, a sport psychologist at Chicago State University, thought that exercise might function similarly to a technique used by some therapists in which they allowed patients to release anxiety by hitting a punching bag.

Kostrubala didn't believe that theory. "That's not true," he asserted. "The person who learns to strike a paper bag may just as easily strike someone else, because that's what he's trained to do" (Higdon, 1978, p. 38).

Kostrubala, then living in San Diego amidst a substantial number of runners, had made certain observations about runners and running. "I have talked to many runners, runners who run long, medium, and short distances," he said, "and I have come to the conclusion that running done in a particular way is a form of natural psychotherapy. It stimulates the unconscious and is a powerful catalyst to the individual psyche."

During the same period (the late 1970s), Robert S. Brown, MD, an enthusiastic runner himself, worked as a psychiatrist at the University of Virginia. He administered psychological tests to university students who took part in various athletic programs. His findings were quite revealing.

We showed that there is some anti-depressant effect with a sport that is not too vigorous, such as girls' softball. There is much *more* therapeutic value in something more active, like girls' basketball or tennis. But as for maximum results, jogging seems to offer the most sustained improvements. Jogging shows very measurable changes in depression levels before and after. Even people who score normal on the depression scale become even more normal as they become physically fit. (Higdon, 1978, p. 36)

Another pioneer of that period who has continued to explore the curative powers of exercise is William P. Morgan, a psychologist at the University of Arizona. One study cited by Morgan involved 100 professors at the University of Missouri. The professors took psychological tests before they embarked on a fitness program involving jogging, swimming, cycling, and weight lifting. "All of those who showed depression in psychological testing before the six-week program had a reduction in the level of depression by exercising," Dr. Morgan stated (Higdon, 1978, p. 36). Morgan found similar results when he studied prisoners in Wisconsin and police officers in Texas.

But even Morgan was skeptical about identifying the mechanism that was at work. "But *why* is it good for you?" he asked. "If it's good because of some time-out factor, that's one matter. If it's because of cell adaption, that's another" (p. 38).

The "time-out factor" Morgan referred to was his theory that the good effects of physical activity may come not directly from the activity itself, but rather from the fact that the stressed person took some time out from that stress to be in a more peaceful environment, thereby creating a sort of protective parcel within a very stressful situation.

Morgan's time-out theory came as the result of an experiment done at the University of Wisconsin by a doctoral candidate under his charge. The experiment involved three groups: The first group exercised, the second group learned to meditate, and the third (the control group) merely sat around in comfortable chairs during the same time period in a sound-filtered room. All three groups showed noticeable reductions in anxiety, hence Morgan's conclusion that the key factor might well be the time spent away from the real-world anxiety-producing situations. Kostrubala felt the time-out factor was nonsense.

That's peanuts! If you're only curing mild forms of anxiety, you're not getting at the roots of true mental illness. Besides, there's a funny value in our society that says anxiety is bad, and that's not true. Some anxiety is absolutely essential for survival in our society. And some depression is necessary too. If you go around with an absolutist notion saying that all anxiety is bad, all paranoia is bad, and all these symptoms are pathological conditions, you're missing the boat. There are many more serious mental conditions prevalent in society today, and in many cases long-distance running can provide some stunning cures, much more than most traditional psychiatrists today are willing to admit. (Higdon, 1978, pp. 38-39)

The mechanism causing the improvements was still being sought, as were larger study groups.

Carlos J.G. Perry, MD, interviewed for *The Physician and Sportsmedicine* in the mid-1970s, told of gaining increased respect from a paranoid patient with whom he had begun to play handball. Although Perry indicated that the camaraderie developed on the court might have been a partial answer, he suspected there was something more. "I think some chemical mediator is involved," he said. "Some chain of biochemical events is caused by the exercise" (Higdon, 1978, p. 39). Perry's surmise turned out to be quite astute. Subsequent research on endorphin release instigated by exercise would provide his theories with validity.

While all this was going on, however, John H. Greist of the University of Wisconsin was posting warnings against assuming that physical activity would help in all psychological cases. Despite favorable results obtained when he put patients into running programs, Greist was justifiably and logically wary of using running for severely depressed patients.

> I think it is possible that an emphasis on running as a treatment for depression at this time, without proper understanding of its limitations as well as its benefits, could actually be dangerous to many depressed individuals. It seems highly probable that the most seriously depressed individuals will not respond to running. These individuals are often suicidal (80 percent of the approximately 50,000 suicides per year come from this group) and a failure to improve from a highly touted 'running therapy' might well be the sort of failure that could lead to a suicide attempt. (Higdon, 1978, pp. 40-41)

During the mid-1970s, Dr. Brown of the University of Virginia organized a search for answers as to why he felt euphoric when he ran, and why the same seemed to be true of some 2,000 subjects he studied psychologically before and after exercise. "I've demonstrated to my satisfaction that not just exercise, but athletic-type training will reduce both anxiety and depression at the highly significant level statistically," he said (p. 41).

At that point, hoping to find out *why* this happened, he began working with Fred Goodwin, MD, at the National Institutes of Mental Health (NIMH) in Bethesda, Maryland. The NIMH was one of only two labs in the country at that time that could measure neurotransmitter metabolites. Tests of blood and urine taken from subjects at intervals of 1, 2, and 3 hours after exercise clearly showed the presence of an antidepressant factor about 2 hours after the exercise was completed. Unfortunately, at that time Brown and Goodwin were unable to identify the chemical factors involved. Brown speculated:

> When you run a mile and feel better, is it salt loss? Is it a neurotransmitter change? Is it hyperthermia? Is it all these things, or just what?

Certainly to me, as a psychiatrist, it's certainly more than a psychological phenomenon. It's a biological phenomenon too. (p, 42)

The experiments caused Brown to forever change his methods of treating patients.

> In the past, where I would use antidepressant pills the way a trainer might pass out salt tablets, now I hardly ever use them. I now take an in-depth exercise inventory of a patient with the same kind of interest that I once took a sexual history. I talk with my patients, and I jog with them. Until this point, it has been mostly a subjective demonstration, but we hope to demonstrate it objectively soon. (p. 42)

The mid-1970s, then, were a turning point for groundbreaking in the area of psychological factors involved in aerobic exercise. The period was also significant because of the suspicions that were raised regarding the existence of some chemical reaction or reactions to sustained aerobic exercise. The chemical reaction that was involved centered on an opiate called beta-endorphin that is produced by the brain.

HOW ENDORPHINS WORK

The chemical within the body that scientists in the 1970s were searching for—the substance that accounted for the runner's high and that made a seemingly boring activity pleasurable and addictive—was isolated near the middle of that decade.

James Hughes (1975), a research professor at Marischal College in England, was studying addictive drugs. He and his colleagues, among them Hans Kosterlitz of the University of Aberdeen, Scotland, discovered that the human body has the capacity to manufacture its own drugs in the opiate family. Subsequent research has further isolated three such opiates: endorphins, enkephalins, and dynorphins.

As Patrick J. Bird (1987) reported in an article on the runner's high, exercise-related research has concentrated on the endorphins. The endorphins are morphine-like chemicals produced by some portions of the brain, the pituitary gland, and nearby tissue.

David C. Nieman explained it this way in his book *The Sports Medicine Fitness Course* (1986):

> The body has an amazing, recently-discovered hormonal system of morphine-like chemicals called 'endogenous opioids.' These are of interest because their receptors are found in the hypothalamus and limbic systems of the brain, areas associated with emotion and behavior. Endogenous opioids such as beta-endorphin have been associated with decrease of pain, increase of memory, and regulation of appetite, sex, blood pressure, and ventilation.

During exercise, the pituitary increases its production of beta-endorphin, with the result that its concentration rises in the blood. Several laboratories, including our own here at Loma Linda University have now measured this increase of beta-endorphin with exercise. Some researchers now speculate that exercise of high enough intensity may open up the blood-brain barrier, allowing access of the beta-endorphin from the blood into the brain, helping to decrease pain, elevate mood, and decrease feelings of fatigue. In addition, beta-endorphin appears to discourage the normal exercise-induced rise in adrenaline and noradrenaline which may make the exerciser feel better. (pp. 254-255)

Some scientists (including Kostrubala) have theorized that the body's ability to produce its own opiates to reduce pain is an ancient system that fostered the survival of the species by allowing prehistoric man to keep hunting for food despite slight injuries and general discomforts resulting from the previous hunt. Once the hunter's body was warmed up and the endorphins began flowing, the aches and pains were alleviated, and the hunt could proceed almost as though the hunter were completely healthy. The fact that the endorphins also bestowed a feeling of equanimity during the activity may have caused the hunter to see the hunt as pleasurable, thereby perpetuating it—and by that means, perpetuating the tribe's existence.

Much of the recent laboratory work to isolate the natural opiates has benefited exercise researchers through a left-handed logic. Hughes's identification of the opiates resulted from research funded for the study of addictive drugs.

Another similar study is ongoing at Stanford University under the direction of pharmacologist Avram Goldstein, who is seeking to learn more about the receptors on the surfaces of nerve cells and how they receive and react to morphine and other drugs.

The body manufactures opiate-like substances that are picked up by the receptors on nerve endings, many of them in or near the brain. These opiates alleviate pain and discomfort while also elevating the mood, not just during the activity but also for several hours afterward. The release of these endorphins (and enkephalins) is stimulated by a variety of events: acupuncture, pain, stress, psychological disturbances (such as schizophrenia and depression), sexual activity, suggestion, and *strenuous physical activity*.

The implications are obvious: A person does not have to go to the local crack or cocaine or heroin dealer in search of a high that is likely to eventually cause a physical and emotional breakdown. Instead of paying thousands of dollars to support a coke habit, that same person can pay $39.95 for a pair of running shoes and enjoy a self-induced high that has a battery of positive physical and psychological by-products: good cardiovascular health, lower blood pressure, muscle tone, weight control, increased self-esteem, and so on.

This high, combined with the factors outlined in the last chapter that tend to encourage an aerobic athlete to keep at it, can literally change a person's life for the good or, taken to extreme, can turn a good habit into a bad addiction.

THE OPIATE OF INSTANT GRATIFICATION

Suppose it were possible to get high once or even twice a day without the damaging effects of the common illegal drugs such as cocaine, crack, heroin, or marijuana. Suppose that this daily high, instead of producing debilitating effects, actually did just the opposite: It conferred general fitness, a feeling of self-esteem, weight control, and myriad other benefits. Suppose this high came about without any dealings with a middleman (dealer or pusher). And further, suppose this high were free.

Such a high seems too good to be true, too outrageous. It seems like a blueprint drawn up by someone designing a utopian world.

Yet, as we've seen, the aerobic lifestyle delivers what was described. It produces a high on a regular basis, it improves the physical and psychological profile of the practitioner, it benefits society by building a healthy person (instead of one bowed over with sicknesses that tax the medical apparatus and the Medicare system), and it benefits the person's family by increasing longevity.

And as we've seen, an aerobic lifestyle also supplies the user with a good deal of that difficult-to-find commodity: instant gratification.

We've seen that the regular aerobic program provides its own coach and cheerleading squad to encourage continued participation by releasing endorphins in the brain that gradually addict the exerciser to the exercise. The endorphin connection comes above and beyond the numerous benefits associated with regular exercise that make it even further addictive.

Unfortunately, there is evidence that addiction to aerobic exercise is not unlike being addicted to any other drug, at least in the way it works.

We have studiously played down, until this point, discussion of what we would call the professional aerobic athlete. And this is for a very good reason.

Since the running revolution of the mid-1970s, discussion of the runner's high has always elicited scorn from professional aerobic athletes. They claim that there is no such thing, that if there *were* such a thing, surely *they* would have experienced it, given the high level at which they pursue their aerobic sports. They have, therefore, consistently written the runner's high off as nonsense and have been less than kind in their evaluations of amateur runners who even mention the term.

With further understanding of the role of endorphins, however, and with more sophisticated means of measuring them, scientists have formulated certain axioms that explain why the professional aerobic athlete who has been running or cycling or swimming competitively for more years than not never experiences the high and why novice runners can and do.

Chan (1986) cited a 1981 study by D.B. Carr in which prolonged training and increased fitness were associated with a leveling off or decline in the production of beta-endorphin the body's natural opiate. "Carr theorized that the more physically fit an individual becomes, the less beta-endorphin is needed in response to the stress of exercise" (p. 431).

This explains why high-level aerobic athletes scoff at the notion of runner's high. The more fit one becomes—and these national- and world-class athletes are at the top of the fitness pyramid—the less the exercising stimulates the release of the beta-endorphins, and therefore the less chance there is for the athlete to experience the high and to become hooked on the exercise itself. For this reason, exercise for many world-class athletes is merely a means to an end—to stellar performances and to earning a living—and many of them are quite candid in saying that when their career is finished, they'll be happy to be done with the constant training, and may never exercise another step as long as they live.

The other significant aspect of research findings concerning beta-endorphin is that the positive addiction to aerobic exercise follows the same profile as the negative drug addictions: A tolerance is built up, and in order to produce the same high, the same effect, more and more exercise is needed as the athlete becomes more competent at the chosen sport.

The analogy of drug addiction is fitting. A drug is typically much more effective for a person whose body is naive to that drug. Thus, a teetotaler who drinks an ounce of whiskey will be much more profoundly affected than a regular drinker who takes the same amount. The regular drinker will hardly feel the effects, while the alcohol-naive teetotaler will most likely be reeling.

The more of a drug a person regularly ingests, the greater quantities of that drug are eventually needed to produce a significant effect. The body builds up a tolerance to the drug if it is constantly administered at lower levels.

The same pattern holds for the aerobic athlete. The more fit the athlete becomes, the more the beta-endorphins are shut down. The typical response, then, would be to do more and more exercise to get the same pleasant effect that the athlete received when the body was exercise-naive.

Chan (1986) has stated it quite simply:

Many individuals reported the need to exercise daily and for longer periods of time to achieve the same feelings of relaxation, achievement, and satisfaction that less exercise had previously produced. . . .

In other words, an athlete may need to run or exercise longer, harder, or faster to maintain antidepressant and antianxiety effects. (pp. 429, 431)

The amateur aerobic athlete caught up in the positive addiction to exercise is then faced with a choice between two alternatives:

1. Exercise more and more until the beta-endorphins are stimulated less and less and exercising is more like a job than like fun, or
2. Exercise more and more until the body breaks down and becomes chronically or traumatically injured.

For most amateur aerobic athletes, who have not built up to their current level of fitness in a slow, methodical way, but who have rather pushed, pushed, pushed it, the latter of the two alternatives is only too common.

THE WALKING WOUNDED: TOO MUCH TOO SOON

The need to do more athletically in order to get the same chemical (endorphin) satisfaction as the body becomes more and more fit sets the aerobic athlete up for trouble and leads, ultimately, to only one end: injury.

Coaches of well-trained, long-term aerobic athletes subscribe to the training theory that the burden of training should never be increased more than 5 percent per year. For many coaches, one of the most difficult chores is not motivating young athletes but reining them in so that they do not prematurely burn out. Bill Dellinger, track coach at the University of Oregon, trained Alberto Salazar. Salazar was the type of kid who would train to exhaustion every day if allowed to do so. One of Coach Dellinger's hardest tasks was to make certain that Alberto did not sneak out on his own and train beyond what was written into the schedule. To the elite athlete, too much training can be much more devastating than too little.

The wisdom of increasing the training load by only 5 percent per year for national- and world-class athletes came after many years of trial and error. But the wisdom has been proven over and over.

Unfortunately, most of the aerobic athletes swelling the starting fields at races in the late 1970s and early 1980s were anything but well-trained. Some of them had never been athletic in their lives; others had not been athletic for a decade or two. Under those circumstances, the wise approach would have been to increase the training load by less than 5 percent per year so that the body could adapt gradually to the demands being placed upon it.

But, these amateur aerobic athletes had no coaches to rein them in. They went out and trained on their own, trained with vague ideas of what to do, trained from advice given to them by other amateurs who had been at it only a few months longer than they had. It was not uncommon for a person who had not exercised in a decade to take up running and 9 months later run a marathon. I'm afraid I was one of them.

Hindsight is a wonderful perch from which to evaluate actions. If I had it to do over again, I'd have waited literally years after getting back into running until I ran a marathon. But it was easy to get caught up in the "running movement," in the excitement. Thousands of Americans who had never run a step in their lives got into running, trained like crazy, ran a marathon, beat themselves up, trained again, and ran another and another and another. And in the meantime made podiatrists and ortho-pedic surgeons rich.

It is worth taking a moment to examine the order in which the body gets fit. There are three basic stages, involving different body systems:

1. *Cardiovascular system.* The primary benefit from an aerobic lifestyle goes to the heart, lungs, and blood vessels. Cardiovascular fitness usually comes about within the first 2 months of a regular aerobic program. Between 45 and 60 days after the start of such a program, the heart and lungs have made major improvements. The evidence is in the ease (compared to the first day of working out) with which the athlete can run a mile.

2. *Muscles.* Beyond the early—and lasting—benefits to the heart muscle, other muscles take somewhat longer to get used to the demands made on them by an aerobic fitness program. The heart muscle has an advantage: It is pumping (and therefore in use) 24 hours a day no matter what the individual is doing, so it has some-thing of a jump on other muscles. Muscle tissue takes time to be-come toned, and to reach a level of being toned, it must be flexible. As we age, muscle tissue becomes less and less flexible. A fitness program inflicted on a 40-year-old body will gradually add muscle strength and some muscle toning, but some muscle tissue will never become well toned because the aging process—combined with disuse—has stiffened the tissue. Additionally, it is very easy—especially for the inexperienced exerciser—to stress muscles, which further hinders their proper development. Even an extremely care-ful exerciser will find that it can take a year or more to bring some of the larger muscles around to the point where they are toned. Because of aging and disuse, some muscle tissue will never be revived.

3. *Joints, tendons, cartilage, bone.* Aging and disuse causes tendons and cartilage to dry out, to become inflexible and brittle. They also cause the lubricating sacs in the joints to dry up. And they cause the bones to lose mineral content, especially calcium, thereby making them brittle and prone to cracking and breaking. The problem with these

areas is that they are not infused with blood vessels as are the major body organs and the muscles, where the blood vessels provide the route for tissue repair and/or tissue building. An exercise program may bring the heart and lungs around quickly and may eventually bring the muscles around, but the joints, tendons, cartilage, and bones can take years to turn around. Granted, a regular, judicious exercise program will eventually improve the flexibility of the tendons and the cartilage, it will gradually cause the joints to become lubricated (very gradual use of the joints stimulates the lubricating sacs to function again), and it will gradually improve bone density. But it is a mighty slow process. And the older you are, the slower the process. It can literally take years and years for the joints and the bones and the tendons and cartilage to catch up to the heart, lungs, and muscles.

If the joints and bones are not exercised gently and given the time they need to come around, they are going to cause problems—very severe problems.

Which brings us to a key word in the lexicon of the millions of aerobic athletes in the world: *overuse.*

There are several types of injuries that the human body can suffer. A person suffers a broken leg in a traffic accident and it's called a traumatic injury. Grandpa broke his leg 50 years ago, but for the last 10 years it's given him nothing but problems, and we call it a chronic injury. If Uncle Joe takes up running at 40 and, within a year, suffers a stress fracture of the lower leg, it's called an overuse injury.

Uncle Joe's problem came not from a violent, traumatic insult to his leg, but from a gradual wearing down caused by running thousands of steps every day for a year. The bone, assaulted every day in the same manner, with the same stresses being fed along the same lines, just couldn't take it any longer, and it cracked.

Some poetically inclined doctors call overuse injuries the injuries of excellence, meaning that the victim broke a leg (suffered a stress fracture) while pursuing a better body through exercise. No matter what euphemism one uses, however, the guy's got a broken leg, plain and simple.

Overuse injuries are simply due to the athlete's doing too much too soon. The mind is willing to do more, but the body is incapable of obliging.

The less athletic background a person brings to the aerobic sport, the more biomechanical problems the person is likely to have. Also, the greater the person's tendency to become addicted to the sport, the more likely he or she is to suffer overuse injuries.

An aerobic athlete need not be addicted to suffer an overuse injury. Aerobic athletes who faithfully heed Cooper's 20 minutes a day, 3 or 4 days a week, can suffer an overuse injury just as an addicted runner can. The addicted runner, however, is more likely to suffer the overuse injury, the injury is likely to be more serious, and the athlete is more likely to compound the problem by attempting to train through it. The addicted athlete is inspired to continue training even if there is a hint of an oncoming injury and, because of the compulsion fed by the addiction, is more likely to attempt to train through aches and pains, thereby causing more aches and pains.

The problem, as we saw in the previous section, is further complicated by the fact that the more effort the athlete puts in and the better shape the athlete gets into, the more exercise is needed to produce the same endorphin stimulation that came from a relatively meager workout a year before.

Just as the heroin addict will take chances that a straight person would never contemplate in order to get the next fix, so the addicted aerobic athlete will do workouts that defy all common sense in an attempt to get the aerobic fix. This extends to gambling with possibly crippling injuries just to get in the next run or to keep a string of workouts unbroken.

Podiatrists and orthopedic surgeons, in treating long-distance runners who have suffered stress fractures, routinely place an injured limb in a cast when the extremity would heal without one. They do this in an attempt to prevent the athlete from continuing to train on the stress fracture. From experience they know that if they do not immobilize the injured bone the runner will be out running on it in a few days, injuring it further.

It is not uncommon for an injured athlete, after being immobilized for a week, to go to the hardware store and buy a hacksaw to cut the cast off because the athlete cannot stand to go any longer without working out. It is also not uncommon for the athlete to then further aggravate the stress fracture, turning it into a more serious, possibly debilitating bone break.

This obsession with getting in the workout no matter what is clearly a sign of addiction. When the importance of the workout transcends consideration for the injured body part, the addiction has reached serious proportions: The athlete has gone beyond both commitment and common sense, and is being driven by an irrational force.

Commitment means long-term involvement. It implies a genuine love of the activity and a dedication that would override anything that would prevent participation in it. Running on a foot that is suffering from a stress fracture flies in the face of common sense; it undermines commitment to the activity because it is a short-term approach ignoring potentially serious consequences that could easily prevent the athlete from ever running again.

Only those who have taken leave of their senses or who have become negatively addicted would continue to train on a broken leg. There is only one outcome to such madness, and that is further injury.

Yet, in typical junkie fashion, those who *do* train on broken bones see themselves as heroic or as martyrs who deserve the respect of others. Reality, for these people, has been pushed very, very far away.

When injured, addicted aerobic athletes have pushed their bodies so far that they just cannot physically go another step; the classic reactions of the seriously addicted come thundering in.

The Pain of Withdrawal

For many years American cigarette manufacturers successfully fought the contention that cigarette smoking is addictive. For years the surgeon general wanted cigarette packs to carry a warning against addiction. In mid-1988, Surgeon General C. Everett Koop created storm waves among the cigarette manufacturers by announcing that research findings had demonstrated that nicotine can cause addiction.

Koop's general definition of addiction included four classic characteristics:

1. The substance produces mood-altering effects.
2. The substance promotes consistent and repetitive patterns of use.
3. Continued use may lead to tolerance and the need for increased dosage.
4. Cessation of use leads to withdrawal symptoms, including: irritability, poor concentration, and sleep disturbance.

This outline of classic addiction seems to be a framework that would readily fit aerobic addiction:

1. Mood-altering effects are produced, both psychologically and physiologically, during the course of a regular aerobic program.
2. Consistent and repetitive patterns of use are essential to an aerobic program, and growing addiction to the activity promotes even more consistency and locks one into repetitive patterns.
3. The more efficient the aerobic athlete becomes, the less of a high is generated; this causes the athlete to do more to gain the same effect.
4. Cessation of the aerobic activity, whether through injury or through choice, produces classic withdrawal symptoms.

Chan and Grossman published a study called "Psychological Effects of Running Loss on Consistent Runners" (1988). These authors cited the rather voluminous studies defining the positive psychological changes brought on by a regular running program. They then examined "directly the psychological and emotional effects of running loss for consistent runners who were unable to run because they were injured" (p. 876).

What is especially startling with this study is that the subjects (60 runners, 32 women and 28 men) were not what many, myself included, would consider highly addicted runners. The group consisted of runners between 15 and 50 years of age, who ran at least three times a week for a minimum of a year, and who ran more than 20 miles a week when not injured. Runners at those levels would be considered by many to be only moderately addicted, if at all. Yet the study's subjects tended to exhibit the classic symptoms.

The subjects were divided into two groups, the first comprising 30 runners who "were unable to run for a period of four weeks following a running-related injury." Chan and Grossman called this group the *prevented runners*. The second group of 30 runners, labeled *continuing runners*, served as the control group; they were not injured and were able to maintain their running mileage.

Each runner was given a "running information" questionnaire (dealing primarily with demographic information and running background) and three standardized psychological scales used to measure self-esteem, depression, and mood state. The tests were the Rosenberg Self-Esteem Scale (Rosenberg, 1965), the Zung Depression Scale (Zung, 1965), and the Profile of Mood States (POMS) (McNair, 1971).

Results of the study indicated that the injured subjects who were prevented from running were suffering significantly greater overall psychological distress than the runners who were still active. Also, the prevented runners reported greater overall disturbance of mood; exhibited significantly more tension, anxiety, depression, confusion, anger, and hostility; and had less vigor than their still-running counterparts. The prevented runners reported significantly lower self-esteem than the control group; they also reported greater dissatisfaction with their body image.

Chan and Grossman concluded that "our group of runners who were prevented from running reported symptoms commonly noted in withdrawal from addictions such as depression, over-all mood disturbance, and decreased self-esteem" (p. 881).

Although the objective of the study was to test the psychological effects of running deprivation, the researchers, in their conclusions, also made an observation about the possible chemical involvement: "A sudden discontinuation of a running regimen could result in changes in endorphin levels, which might help to explain our prevented runners' mood disturbances and other symptoms of stress" (p. 882).

The withdrawal symptoms and the accompanying feelings of depression and lowered self-esteem would seem to conspire against the addicted runner. To avoid these unpleasant consequences, the addicted runner might choose to run with or through injuries.

In the bigger picture, however, the psychological and physical symptoms of addiction can tend to set the individual up for a grand disillusionment with the aerobic activity itself, especially if the injury lasts for any great length of time (long enough to cause the benefits of fitness to evaporate) or if the injury is such that it either will be permanent or will take months or years to correct itself.

It is not unusual for the formerly committed and addicted athlete to metamorphose from the sport's biggest booster to its biggest critic when denied the soothing effects of the activity. And because the critic is a former practitioner and not merely a sideline observer, the criticisms take on added weight.

This scenario happened to one of the biggest boosters of the sport of long-distance running I'd ever met. Phil Lenahan consistently ran sub-3-hour marathons, frequently competed in ultramarathon events (he ran the first annual Cow Mountain 50-miler with me after spending months talking me into training for longer events), regularly traveled to Boston to compete in the country's premier marathon, and in fact gravitated toward a job that in part included promoting running races. Yet when he suffered a leg injury that hobbled him for well over a year, he became an embittered and vocal critic of the sport. Fortunately, his injury resolved itself and Lenahan eased himself back into running, but at a level much more healthy from a psychological point of view. When I ran into him at the starting line of the San Jose Half-Marathon several years ago, he had lowered his sights somewhat and was running more for fun than for existence. His good humor and ready smile had returned, although he still tended to tell the same jokes he'd been telling several years before. It was good to have Phil back.

Through the intervention of his serious injury, Lenahan was given the opportunity to reevaluate his running and, when he restarted it, to place it in a different context. He once again considers himself committed to running, but he is not necessarily addicted.

We have seen that the benefits of aerobic activity can conceal the trap of potential addiction. Now we will consider how to regulate a fitness program to prevent the negative aspects of addiction (chapter 5), and then consider what can be done to bring an aerobic athlete back to an even keel if the threshold of addiction has already been crossed (chapter 6).

5
CHAPTER

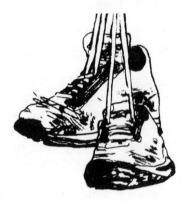

HOW TO MANAGE FITNESS TO PREVENT ADDICTION

An overly simplistic way to avoid the pitfalls of exercise addiction—and they can be many—would be just to avoid involvement in all types of endurance activities. This is very easy to do, as millions of sedentary Americans prove every day.

To do nothing, however, is to passively accept the philosophy that what will be, will be. Certainly not a classic American reaction to life, but unfortunately a reaction that is becoming classic for too many who still seem to feel that since heart disease is the number one killer of Americans, it must be number one for a good reason, and what can be done about a disease that's formed a dynasty, anyway? In actuality, heart disease is the greatest killer of Americans by default. It is a disease of passivity, a silent killer that grows as moss grows—on an unrolling stone.

Even minor breaks in that pattern of passivity can produce significant results. A regular program of brisk walking 4 to 5 days a week exercises the heart muscle enough to—excuse the pun—make great strides against the creeping incursion of heart disease.

GOVERNING THE EXERCISE ADDICTION

It would be easy for the passionately passive to roll down their sleeves and declare that they're going to do their part to avoid the injuries and burnout of exercise addiction by doing nothing. But the passionately passive aren't likely to be reading this book. The person curious about the exercise fix is more likely the person contemplating an aerobic fitness program, already involved in one, considering expanding one, or already getting perhaps too involved in one.

For these active people, here are some simple guidelines for keeping endurance sports under control, at whatever level they are pursued. The suggestions are presented as a series of governors—mechanisms to restrict speed so the exerciser does not career out of control.

Stay Within the Bounds of Cooper's Program

For people who are contemplating getting into aerobic fitness for their own good, or who are already involved in a modest sense, the best way to avoid exercise addiction is to keep the exercise modest.

Do your exercise routine regularly 3 to 4 days a week, but keep it to 20 minutes or less each session and keep your goals focused on only the health benefits. Follow guidelines and workouts as outlined in Cooper's aerobics program. Keep the exercise sensible; don't let friends persuade you to train for the local 5K race "because it will be fun to do." If you start training for the local 5K, you *may* train above and beyond the 20 or 25 minutes that confer health and fitness benefits. Everything beyond that is done for its own sake or for your own satisfaction. Fitness at that point can become contagious and make you want more of it, which leads to more and more training and can ultimately lead to problems.

Thousands of busy executives, for whom time is a rare and precious commodity, maintain successful fitness programs of 20 minutes at a time, 3 to 4 days a week. Generally inspired by Cooper, they have been able by sticking to this modest program to improve their health markedly without succumbing to the lure of doing more. The governor on their motors, of course, is their very lack of leisure time. They have seen the importance of exercise to improve health and have carefully scheduled into their busy days the habit of getting that health through exercise.

A tendency toward moderation in exercise, based on the abundant (and constantly growing) proof that a little is enough to improve health, is beginning to invade most health clubs throughout the country. The hardcore exerciser has frequently crashed and burned, and a more sensible and sane approach to exercise for health is growing.

It is imperative, then, to adhere to your goals of exercising strictly for health. Keep foremost in your mind that the reason you are *investing* that 20 minutes a day 3 to 4 days a week is to improve your chances of *not* becoming one of the 738,000 Americans who die of some form of heart disease each year. Keep your strong commitment to regular exercise in perspective: It is a prophylactic, not unlike brushing your teeth to prevent cavities or regularly checking the brakes on your car. Under no circumstances should you allow your exercise to escalate to the point that it consumes all of your ''free'' time.

If Build You Must, Do So at a Slow, Logical Pace

For those who *do* exercise not only for health reasons—that is, who go *beyond* Cooper—keeping four specific cautions in mind can prevent a headlong rush into the trap of exercise addiction:

Build slowly. This may seem overly simplified and too obvious to state, but it is one of the most easily forgotten precepts of fitness. It is easily forgotten, first, because Americans tend to be very impatient and, second, because once an exerciser allows the program to progress a mite faster, the momentum begins to pull both the exerciser and the program along by subtly greater degrees until the whole program is out of control. What is meant by out of control? The program dictates to the exerciser instead of the other way around.

When an exercise program is kept modest, it is taken somewhat lightly. The exerciser stays committed to it, but the time needed to fulfill that commitment is insubstantial and fits easily into a daily routine. It can become as second nature as brushing the teeth first thing in the morning. However, once goals are upgraded, once an exercise program is allowed to expand, it has a sort of incursion effect, like a soft spot in an apple. Little by little it consumes more time each day, but it provides such rewards—both immediate and long term—that it is not only tolerated but gladly accommodated.

The barrage of good things happening—growth in self-esteem, weight control, increased energy reserves immediately following exercise, increased muscle tone, and so on—escalates the desire for more. Soon the exerciser is setting racing goals, pushing the program along at a rate that may feel satisfying but is not especially wise or beneficial for other body systems that cannot necessarily keep up the pace.

When you build slowly and with control, no body part suffers, and both body and mind can perceive the exercise program as a pleasant adjunct instead of a new passion—and possible stressor.

Get a checkup. Building slowly is essential for good, sane development of the cardiovascular system of anyone over 35. If you're under 35 and not grossly out of shape, this is of less concern. A relatively healthy person under 35 who has no history of abnormalities in the heart, arteries, or lungs should be able to embark on a fairly ambitious endurance exercise program if tried and true training methods are followed and workloads increased logically. For the person 35 or older, both a medical checkup and a stress test are advisable. This point is repeated again and again, but just as you wouldn't drive cross country without first checking over your car's basic operating systems, you should not start on an endurance fitness program without first being cleared medically. Your body's worth more than the family car, after all, and should be treated with at least as much respect and care.

The cardiovascular system is the body system that tends to respond first to an endurance program. A person beginning an endurance fitness program experiences some initial discomfort in attempting to reverse the effects of a sedentary lifestyle. But within a 2-month period this should begin to change. If the program is followed regularly, breathing becomes easier. Conversation can actually be maintained during exercise. This comfort area increases if the exercise program is kept constant and not escalated. Many exercisers, upon reaching the comfort level, maintain a program at that plateau. This is wise because it allows the third caution to catch up.

Recognize your limitations. Although the cardiovascular system responds quickly to endurance style exercise, the same is not true of the muscles, joints, ligaments, and other body parts more mechanically oriented. As a person ages the bones become more brittle, the joints less flexible, and the muscles less able to perform efficiently. Starting an endurance exercise program—especially if one is 35 or over—does not reverse these characteristics overnight. After several years of regular exercise, improvements in these systems *will* happen, but a person cannot turn on a spigot and have them all at once just because the cardiovascular system is more efficient.

The fact that many other body systems take considerably longer to get fit than does the cardiovascular system accounts for the alarming injury rate among overly enthusiastic, impatient exercisers. The cardiovascular system is willing, but the joints are weak—hence, the inordinate number of injuries in the knees of runners; the shoulders of swimmers; the backs and necks of bicyclists; and the shins, ankles, Achilles tendons, and feet of runners. Too much too soon quickly finds the weak points in the anatomy and lays waste to them, often foreshortening a fitness career that could have bestowed incredible rewards upon a person.

During the running revolution of the late '70s, many very enthusiastic runners never made it out the other side. They dropped out from chronic injuries brought on as they escalated their programs too high too soon. The lure of the marathon destroyed the running career of many an impatient American. Only an adding machine could enumerate the foolish who saw marathoning as the "in" thing. Feeling compelled to be with whatever was in, they trained for a marathon as their first—and, ultimately, last—road race. A sad commentary on terminal impatience.

In an endurance program that is built slowly and carefully, the muscles, joints, bones, and ligaments are given time to catch up with and keep abreast of the cardiovascular advances. This creates a balanced organism instead of a strong set of lungs on a rickety set of legs.

Prepare yourself emotionally. Psychologically and emotionally it is better to build slowly because too much change at once can disrupt a person's life balance. Any major life change is disruptive to psychological balance, and changing from a butterball to a marathoner in one year can be a major blow to a person's psychology. Although the change can be filled with good feelings and impressions, it is nonetheless a change that represents a loss of the way things were. As such it ranks right there with the loss of a loved one or a major career change. And later in life, these psychological changes are harder to handle than they are at a younger, more psychologically pliable age.

The slow, *steady* approach to growth in fitness offers all the benefits while minimizing the shock effect. One can savor the changes and the improvements and take them in stride, fitting them gradually into the rest of one's life.

Major disruptions brought on by changes in the body and the self-perception are accompanied by changes in routine that are necessary to keep those physical changes coming. Although this severely tries the person experiencing the changes, it can be trying for others as well. Family and friends are frequently expected to react positively to such changes, even though the changes are not originating with them or through their decisions but are being literally thrust upon them. They may be going through major psychological change themselves and may lack the extra psychological or emotional energy to deal with something that is—literally—out of their hands and their control. It is a tribute to the American family that so many of them survived one member of the household suddenly becoming fanatical about fitness.

In summary, building a fitness program slowly and almost imperceptibly will have minimum adverse effects upon the exerciser and upon the people with whom he or she interacts every day. And it will discourage exercise addiction, because addiction does not thrive in an environment of slow, steady, patient growth. Instead, it thrives on momentum and rapidly escalating, almost desperate goals.

Periodically Take Time to Review Your Fitness Program

Another way to keep exercise addiction at bay is to schedule periodic reviews and evaluations of your endurance program, during which you set your next modest and realistic short-term goals. Couple this regularly scheduled evaluation with keeping a faithful journal (similar to a diary) of your fitness efforts. Remember to include space for notations on daily occurrences and feelings (see pp. 102-103).

A daily journal records your progress, provides an accurate source of information when it comes time to review your program, and ensures at least one 10-minute period when you remove yourself from your exercising as you objectively evaluate your day. It's especially useful for those with loftier training goals.

A journal entry needn't be complex or time-consuming. Running, triathlon, and cycling diaries or journals are available commercially, but yours can be as simple as a three-by-five card for each day. Put the date in the upper left, then fill the card with information pertinent to your workout(s) that day: time of day, distance run, swum, or cycled; duration of workout; effort (subjectively evaluated) required to do workout; resting pulse rate at rising and at bedtime, some notes on the weather conditions during the workout; a sentence or two summarizing the workout (*Midway through the 4-mile workout, I seemed to hit another gear and the second half was wonderfully exhilarating after a lackluster start.*), a sentence describing your emotional state at the start and completion of the workout; and perhaps a note or two on any other significant events of the day, whether receiving a letter from a long-lost friend or attending a productive meeting with the boss.

Keeping a journal has many advantages:

• It records your life—or at least the part of it that you are sufficiently interested in to comment on every day.

• If you become injured in your pursuit of endurance fitness, it may be possible to backtrack through the journal to discover what preceded that caused the injury. Most overuse injuries, for example, occur between 1 and 2 weeks following the straw that broke the Achilles tendon. With the ability to trace the cause of an injury, you can avoid that injury in the future.

• Should your training result in some outstanding performances, the journal similarly provides a record of the workouts that led to those performances. This record can form the backbone of a training schedule customized specifically to your body's strengths and weaknesses to maximize your efforts.

With your journal as the primary source of historical perspective on your progress, schedule a half hour once a month (or once every 2 months at the minimum) for reviewing your fitness program. With your workouts in front of you in black and white, you'll be able to note progress and backsliding. But more important, you'll be able to modify any patterns that indicate that you're slipping within range of the tentacles of addiction.

If you've gone to the trouble of creating a logical, sensible fitness program characterized by rational, modest increases in effort, your journal will clearly reflect whether or not you are abiding by the plan. If your sport happens to be running, use graph paper to make a graph of your weekly mileage during the time since your last review. If you do this at every review and save the graphs in a three-ring binder, you'll quickly see any major deviations from the cool-headed, logical growth patterns you started with. Don't let yourself sneak in any additional workouts beyond those you planned for—and don't greatly chastise yourself if you've fallen a little short. In the matter of addiction and fitness, falling a little short is much preferable to going overboard.

If your review and evaluation reveal that you have erred on the side of too much exercise, design your next month's schedule to bring it gradually back into pace. Don't make radical cuts over the next week to get back down to where you should be; extend the necessary cuts over a month so that you do not greatly disturb the texture and pace of your workouts.

By taking the time to examine what you are actually doing in the real world workouts—as opposed to the paper programs you've laid out for

My Daily Fitness Diary (Sample)

Date _Mar_ _16_ 19 _89_ _Thu_
　　 month   date 　　 year day

Morning pulse rate _52_ beats per minute; time out of bed _6:30_ a.m.

Workout #1: Type/time of workout _run / 9 a.m._

　　　　　　　 Total time _50:15_ Total distance _7 mi_

Weather/temperature _rainy, overcast / 44°_

Comments on workout _Felt stiff during first 2 miles._
Began to open up gradually. Legs became loose after
going up Crystal Springs Rd. Picked it up on final mile.

Workout #2: Type/time of workout _bike_

　　　　　　 Total time _1:20:32_ Total distance _21 mi_

Weather/temperature _clearing / 57°_

Comments on workout _Kept up good pace for most of_
ride but began to lose it coming up Deer Park Rd. at end.
Will have to go easier all around tomorrow.

Upper body workout:
　　 Sit-ups _30_ Push-ups _15_ Chin-ups _3_

　　 Arm curls _100_ Military presses _50_

Work and errands accomplished today:

1. _Sent proposal to Brian_ 　　6. _Called Paul - no answer_
2. _Bills sent to SGP_ 　　　　 7. _misc. - errands_
3. _letters to clients_ 　　　　 8. _Roughed out Ch14-Slipstream_
4. _Called editor on ms_ 　　　 9. _____
5. _Corrections on EIII to DH_ 　10. _____

Bed-time pulse rate _64_ beats per minute; time of retiring _10:30_ p.m.

Additional comments:

Overall day was great! Accomplished nearly
everything I set out to do.

My Daily Fitness Diary

Date _____ ____ 19 ____ ____
      month date   year day

Morning pulse rate _____ beats per minute; time out of bed _____ a.m.

Workout #1: Type/time of workout _____

                Total time _____ Total distance _____

Weather/temperature _____

Comments on workout _____

_____

_____

Workout #2: Type/time of workout _____

                Total time _____ Total distance _____

Weather/temperature _____

Comments on workout _____

_____

_____

Upper body workout:

    Sit-ups _____ Push-ups _____ Chin-ups _____

    Arm curls _____ Military presses _____

Work and errands accomplished today:

1. _____   6. _____

2. _____   7. _____

3. _____   8. _____

4. _____   9. _____

5. _____   10. _____

Bed-time pulse rate _____ beats per minute; time of retiring _____ p.m.

Additional comments:

yourself—you can readily keep yourself in check and out of the pitfalls of addiction. A gradual, logical increase in workout level wards off potential injury, keeps exercising relatively enjoyable, and allows all body systems to become strengthened more evenly.

Faithfully Employ the Hard/Easy Training Method

People bound for burnout through exercise addiction frequently exhibit a startling tendency toward monotony in their training. Once they are able to run 7 miles a day, they tend to run 7 miles a day, day in and day out. They seldom vary their course, and they decrease their distance only if injury prevents them from doing the magic number for that day (they will usually try, however); they increase it as soon as they are physically able.

Nancy Ditz, top US finisher in the 1988 Olympic (women's) marathon, cited a female marathoner who managed to make the 1984 Olympic Trials by religiously doing 20 miles a day: 10 miles in the morning and 10 in the afternoon, always the same course. As this is written, the woman is no longer able to run.

Some beginning runners of my own experience fell into similar traps. They compulsively ran their 7 miles a day, 6 days a week, and then did their long run on Sunday. Never a variation. And invariably, by the time the race came around, they were running wounded and, had they not been so addicted, would have had the common sense not to line up at the starting line. Of course, they *did* line up, and they hobbled across the finish line well off their planned pace.

The human body will consistently become stronger if it is lightly stressed and then rested. It will just as consistently break down if it is stressed and then stressed some more.

The system of stress and rest is called the *hard/easy method*. It is probably the most basic of all training principles. Yet, among addicted aerobic athletes, it is the most frequently ignored. And this despite the fact that the athlete frequently knows the term hard/easy and can explain it to you.

By implementing a hard/easy method of training, endurance athletes assure themselves of more physical fitness, fewer injuries, better race performances, and a more sane training program.

A wise athlete will lay out a training program weeks in advance (except during "down" periods, something the addicted athlete seldom undertakes) and will stick to that program reasonably well, on the basis of the body's response to it. If the program of a distance runner were Monday through Saturday and looked like this:

Mon—10 miles
Tue—10 miles
Wed—10 miles
Thu—10 miles
Fri—10 miles
Sat—10 miles

something would be amiss. There is no easy time. *Easy* does not mean that no training is done that day, but only that it is of a lesser intensity, whether in terms of distance or effort expended.

By being careful to dial easy days into the week's training equation, the wise runner will enhance the enjoyment of training, extend the time between possible injuries, and head off bouts with addiction.

Either Schedule Rest Days or Take Them When Necessary

Rest days, no matter what one hears from compulsive athletes, are important. They are, in fact, often more important than key workout days. A well-placed rest day can prevent injury, can rejuvenate the athlete psychologically, and can insert a breather in the schedule that averts addiction and burnout.

Most athletes who are balanced in their lives look forward to their rest days as days of rebirth—days in the schedule when the battery is allowed to recharge. It is advisable to schedule at least one rest day into the program each week; it is not unheard of for even serious athletes to schedule 2 rest days, especially as they age.

Rest days need not necessarily be days of complete immobility. But they should be days when whatever physical activity is planned has little, if anything, to do with regular training.

Go on a picnic, take a walk in the park, go on that overnight backpacking trip you've been putting off, play touch football or one-on-one basketball.

One Bay Area distance runner I know takes the rest day concept even farther. He schedules 2 separate weeks during the year when he doesn't run a step. Instead, he goes backpacking in the Sierra Nevada for a week at a time. He claims backpacking uses—and builds up—completely different muscles than does running, and the psychological break brings him back to training with a new, refreshed outlook. Oh, by the way, he *does* win marathons on a fairly regular basis, so it must be doing some good.

Regularly Work Out With a Slower Partner

No two people exercise exactly alike. Some people who train together regularly approximate each other's training. But no two people, no matter how frequently or how long they train together, react in exactly the same way to the training.

This is due largely to the fact that, although similarities in physical systems are apparent, each individual is very much unique in abilities. This is why any book on endurance training begins with and expands upon the basics, but concludes by stressing that the exerciser must know his or her body and customize workouts to improve weak points and capitalize on strengths.

In many of the endurance sports it is not unusual to train with others. Often, you train with those who introduced you to your sport in the first place. This tendency to train at least occasionally with partners covers the entire spectrum of talents. Scott Molina sometimes trains with other top-level triathletes. Bill Rodgers works out around the Boston area with friends who approach his level of ability. Cycle racers, perhaps more than most endurance athletes, tend to ride with other cyclists, to get comfortable riding in a pack, to practice slipstreaming (drafting), and to enjoy companionship on long, arduous rides. Women frequently get together on a weekend morning for a group run, both for protection and for support within the group. Many corporations have running or cycling teams, with groups of team members training together over the lunch hour.

As far as some people are concerned, if it weren't for the fact that they had a training partner, they wouldn't work out at all. Some people need a partner to help motivate them to overcome perceived boredom.

In most instances, working out with one or more partners benefits slower participants, who must challenge themselves in order to remain part of the group. Many people involved in endurance sports find that this effort to keep up accounts for great gains in their training and racing and that when they train alone, their inclination to work so hard vanishes. The weakest link in the group is able to demonstrate more endurance than usual when in the presence of the others. Another benefit reported by many people who work out in small groups is a certain energy transmitted within the group.

When just two partners work out together, the weaker one frequently finds that workouts tend to make him or her stronger, while the partner's presence makes the workout less tedious and frequently "lulls" the weaker of the two into performing at a level he or she finds pleasantly surprising once the workout is over.

If the stronger partner is unsympathetic to the physical condition of the other, however, the weaker one may continually feel at a disadvantage, as though always trying to catch up with the partner. In that case, the weaker partner could be discouraged in further pursuit of a fitness lifestyle. This is frequently a problem for couples attempting to train together. Many a novice female runner has been discouraged from further involvement when her "significant other" consistently pushes the pace, chides her for not keeping up, or uses his stronger conditioning as a tool to play out on the roads some problems the pair have been trying to work out at home. For some members of a couple, the person they live with might be the *worst* person in the world to train with.

As a preventive measure against addiction, training with (and at the level of) a slower or less trained partner once or twice a week, or more frequently if possible, can provide a perfect governor to overtraining and can keep the training in perspective. Besides providing a worthwhile service to your friend by offering encouragement and support, you also provide yourself an opportunity to go slower, to smell the roses, to chat while training, and to enjoy the training at a civilized and humane level instead of pushing and being alone with your own motivations to train harder or longer.

Regular training with a partner is not necessarily easy for the person who originally got involved in fitness as a route to escape many of life's travails. Training with a partner can be almost like backsliding, if you perceive it that way.

Yet running, cycling, or cross-country skiing with a person of lesser ability can be refreshing for the seasoned endurance athlete. It tends to recreate many of the early efforts the experienced athlete invested in training to become more knowledgeable and sophisticated. And it can be rewarding for training partners to learn from each other, while also getting to know each other on a level that is rarely achieved in usual social settings.

For the experienced athlete, such training sessions can be an oasis in the middle of a week's training. These sessions normally follow a slower, more civilized pace; they often provide the only real easy days for some people who tend to push the pace too much too often when they train alone.

Workouts with a weaker partner can recharge one's psychological reservoir, a necessity for training well or for making advances in distance or speed. Most significant, however, is the fact that joint workouts break the downward spiral of taking one's sport too seriously. It is difficult to remain single-minded while working out with someone else. The other person provides too many of the distractions that are necessary for putting at least a few days of training a week back into perspective.

To implement this method for warding off addiction and creating a refreshing training environment, you could arrange to train at least once a week with a complete novice. Offer the beginner the benefit of your experience, not as a didactic teacher, but as a friend giving help and encouragement. It is surprising how refreshing the experience can be for even the most experienced exerciser as the partner begins to grow and improve.

When You Reach the Threshold of Pain, Back Off

As discussed previously, pain is your body's way of telling you something is wrong.

A person who trains to the edge of pain and then continues to train and moves willingly farther into pain is unquestionably asking for trouble.

Under extraordinary circumstances, an elite athlete pushing into pain and beyond in competition is admirable. The athlete has probably trained for a great deal of time and dedicated many years of life to a specific competition. Weighing the pros and cons, the athlete decides that pushing through pain is a gamble worth taking: The rewards are worth the risk of suffering injury. We're talking *pain* here, not the *discomfort* associated with certain efforts.

For the dedicated amateur who "heroically" pushes through pain in order to get workouts accomplished, who habitually endures and perpetuates injuries as a regular price of training, there is no excuse. It is a case of abject addiction, and it is to be avoided.

It is, in fact, absurd.

The amateur athlete is frantically, compulsively training because he or she loves the sport and wants to do better in it. Despite this insatiable urge to do better at any cost, the athlete jeopardizes the physical side of him- or herself with no real promise of improvement. To train injured is to train at well under 100 percent of ability and effort, and to complicate the injury while predisposing oneself to more injuries. This is self-defeating, especially when you consider that taking some time off would both heal the injury and provide much-needed rest, which would likely bring the athlete back fresher and stronger than ever. As an example, Derek Clayton's world's best performance in the marathon in 1969 followed a long layoff forced by injuries. Joan Benoit's sterling performances at the 1984 Olympic Trials and the Olympics came in the wake of a layoff forced by injury.

A person who knowingly trains through injury is a person whose logic gear is stuck in neutral.

A great irony is that the dedicated amateur who not only flirts with injuries but knowingly aggravates them by continuing to train is often the person who claims lifelong commitment to the particular sport. It's ironic because the statements are incongruous with the actions. Training into and through an injury is a good way to increase the odds that you'll be unable to live up to the lifelong commitment to your sport.

One rule of thumb, then, to avoid the pitfalls of exercise addiction, is to refuse to send your body up to the pain threshold. Forget the "no pain, no gain" nonsense. It's an antiquated training axiom, and following it is likely to significantly shorten your training and competitive career.

This is not to say that occasionally training to the point of *discomfort* will shorten your career. A good, hard track workout to build leg speed pushes into the region of discomfort.

But a major difference exists between discomfort and pain. Discomfort is a general feeling of being assaulted by several factors at once: tiredness of the limbs, inability of the lungs to pull in enough oxygen to meet current muscle needs, and so on.

Pain, on the other hand, is a very specific sensation indicating that something is wrong: a side stitch, a sharp sensation under the arch of the foot when the foot touches the ground, a red-hot shooting sensation in the shoulder whenever the arm is raised above the head on a swimming stroke, a stabbing sensation in the outside of the right knee when pumping uphill on the bicycle. Pain is easily pinpointed and described by the person suffering it.

Keep in mind that pain is a sign not that you are getting stronger, but that something is being compromised, broken down, injured. And the only possible result of pushing for more pain is further damage to whatever part of the body is sending out the distress signal. It doesn't take a great deal of logic to understand that a body part that suffers pain and is therefore not functioning properly is not going to function well as an integral part of the training organism.

It seems overly simplified and so moronically basic, but—if it hurts, stop using it until it heals. And then, when you start using it again, begin gently, just in case whatever was hurt isn't healed totally.

After all, you're dedicated to your fitness, your fitness comes by way of your body, and you've only got one body. Your first dedication had best be to maintaining as well as possible the moving parts of that body.

Set Short- and Long-Term Goals

The endurance athlete who meticulously sets realistic short- and long-term goals for training and racing is less likely to be caught up in the breakneck pace required to reach exercise addiction.

The process of sitting down with a piece of paper and outlining goals, and then doing research on training and racing that lets you plan a logical training schedule based upon sound advice from the experts, usually subverts excess. When a training schedule is submitted to the harsh reality of black on white, the errors usually become obvious, especially if the schedule is constructed with even the most rudimentary knowledge of at least one of the numerous books written by past masters in the sport.

When a series of short-term goals and one or two long-term goals are constructed and then committed to paper, the relationship between theory and practice is often made clear. Frequently it is the person with only vague, unformed goals who trains to excess. The one who methodically plans an assault on a goal by mapping out the campaign seldom goes off on an unmarked road.

This is not to say that you must define the goals, put together a schedule that will allow you to achieve those goals, *and then stick to them come hell or high water.* The goals and the schedules are guidelines, logical steps you take to arrive at a destination. The good planner always inserts provisions for slight deviations: contingency plans, if you will.

It's safe to say that if your plan is comprehensible to your fellow endurance athletes, then you won't be detoured down a dangerous side road.

Use Year-Long Schedules With Built-In Down Periods

As discussed in the section on building a fitness program slowly to keep it in control, when you allow yourself to become pulled along by the enthusiasm of the moment, to increase momentum without a plan, you risk going overboard because you've set no bounds, put no governors in place.

The best way to control an endurance fitness program and to make provisions for your body to regularly recuperate is to train in cycles.

As already discussed, these cycles should filter all the way down to the daily level: hard/easy or hard/easy/easy. And certainly to the weekly level: a long workout one weekend followed by an easier long run the next weekend, and so on. Cycles should also be considered at the monthly level: 1st week moderate, 2nd week medium hard, 3rd week hard, 4th week easy.

But the most important cycle for any serious athlete is the annual or yearly cycle. Attention to the yearly cycle is vital to the long-term success of an endurance-sport program. The yearly cycle should be thought of as a natural device. In fact, it is as natural as you can get, for it imitates nature's adaptation to a year's passing.

Whether you think of grizzly bears foraging all summer long and then loading up their reserves in the autumn to hibernate through the winter, or you consider planting a gladiola bulb in late fall to see it blossom in June before going dormant for the rest of the year, everything in nature acknowledges the annual cycle.

The cycle is simply one of resource building, growth, fulfillment, and rest.

For the endurance athlete wishing to grow in a sport, to perform well, and to recover well in preparation for another year's growth and competition, the yearly cycle is mandatory. And for the athlete who wants to keep his or her program under control and on a positive course, the yearly cycle is critical.

Since America is geographically situated in a temperate zone, the seasonal changes come in most of the country with some authority. There is little question as to when it's winter in Kansas, spring in Washington, DC, autumn in New England, or summer in Georgia. Some argue that the seasons are almost nonexistent in places like California and Florida, but to anyone who's lived in either location with their eyes open for more than a year, it is apparent that even those areas undergo seasonal change.

It is logical that such sports as open-water swimming and marathoning have ideal seasons. While distance swimmers might do daily workouts in Lake Michigan in July, they're not likely to do the same in January. Major marathons are scheduled in the spring (April) and autumn (October) to take advantage of favorable weather while avoiding the extremes: snow and sleet in January, exhausting heat in July.

Virtually every serious endurance athlete schedules one or more "down" periods within the yearly cycle to allow the body to recover from a season of hard workouts and competition.

Typically, for marathoners, winter is the recuperation period, spring is the building (distance) period, the summer is the sharpening period (with plenty of shorter races thrown in), and autumn is the prime period for unleashing that supreme effort before again going into a recovery phase. Obviously, for the cross-country skier winter is the prime time for competition, and summer is a good time to recuperate. For the triathlete, summer and early autumn are prime time, and winter is for recuperation.

By taking time at year's end to map out your next year's goals and training efforts, you can create a sort of series of pastures, joined by gates, within which you will follow certain training, racing, and recuperation regimens with some flexibility, but beyond which you will not want to wander for fear of straying from the path you've set. Your program provides the fence that keeps you within those well-defined and well-thought-out grazing and growth areas.

And don't forget to include breaks. "Last year I didn't run at all for the month of December," recalled Ditz. "I didn't do anything. We went skiing for a week. Downhill skiing, not cross-country. I didn't do any aerobic exercise. I porked out. I mean, I really enjoyed myself. I think more athletes should do this. Don't write this, though; this is my secret [laughter]. I try to take a month off. I went 18 months once without a break. It was in 1983-84, and I got injured in 1984. It's the only injury I've ever had."

By mapping out your year to create a logical training formula while setting limits for yourself, you'll be training more like the athletes you

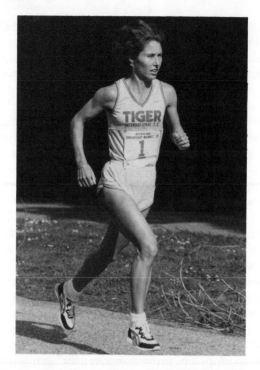

One of three American women to compete in the 1988 Olympic Women's Marathon and the first American woman across the finish line, Nancy Ditz started her running career relatively late in life. She feels that addiction to sports can extend to disciplines outside the aerobic world. She claims her husband is addicted to tennis. (Kenneth Lee photograph)

wish to emulate. And you'll have a tangible tool to keep yourself from straying off the path to your goals and getting lost in a tail-chasing session with addiction.

If You're Injured, Stop!

One sure sign of exercise addiction is when an endurance athlete becomes injured (usually through overuse in training) and continues to train. To a rationally thinking person, that decision to keep on training is at best, illogical, and at worst, downright stupid.

Early in an endurance program, make a pact with yourself that you're engaged in the exercise to benefit yourself in a variety of ways. To hurt yourself is certainly not a goal. Injury and pain do nothing to improve your fitness. So, injury is a sign to stop and pain is a signal to back off until that part of your body heals or stops hurting.

Stopping does not mean completely relinquishing fitness. If you are willing to substitute another endurance sport that maintains your fitness without aggravating your injury, you've come upon a solution. (It is not a solution that a person struck with exercise addiction will easily adapt to, however.)

By laying down a *no training while injured* rule early on, and by applying to that rule the same dedication you're applying to your sensible, moderate growth in fitness, you'll take several giant steps to sidestep the lure of addiction—and ultimately, debilitating injury.

When healing from an injury, remember that you cannot just jump back into training where you left off—you must gradually build back to that level. And remember that although you may feel healed as you take a walk around town, once you resume in your fitness routine, you'll be placing considerably more stress on the injured part than you do while walking. Be careful to ease back into training so that the healing process can continue even as you rekindle your training.

It is a good precaution, when you begin your fitness program, to ask friends who are fit if they know competent professionals who specialize in treating athletic injuries. If treatment is needed, a medical practitioner who engages in some aerobic physical pursuit will be more sympathetic to your predicament.

By consulting a competent professional regarding injuries or suspected injuries, you will take yourself off the hook when you must cut back on exercise or stop it until an injury heals. ''I'm cutting back on training this month on my doctor's recommendation,'' you can tell yourself, and that second opinion can carry a lot of weight with you.

Keep the "Escape" Factor a Healthy Factor

Engaging in an endurance sport as a vehicle of escape from some of the stresses of daily life is not unhealthy and is by no means a sure sign of addiction. An endurance sport used as a daily minivacation from stresses and strains is a commendable coping mechanism for the human mind and body working its way through an increasingly complex world.

Do, however, attempt to keep the escape factor in perspective. If every run or every open-water swim or every Saturday morning bicycle ride is an escape from something, your method of escape may be reaching an unhealthy level.

Unfortunately, it is not so easy to lay out guidelines for this gray area because those of us pursuing an endurance sport bring to it our own psychological package. The role of exercise in the total scheme of dealing with problems is an area where each of us must be brutally honest with ourselves before, during, and after workouts.

Although an endurance sport is a wonderful method of solving problems and of—at least temporarily—avoiding a difficult or painful situation, it should not be substituted for the rational solutions to the problems confronting you. If you run or cycle or swim long distances to get away from something, some problem, and you never come back from the workout with the refreshing feeling that now you're ready to tackle the problem, that you've gotten a new perspective on it, or that it has suddenly proved to be less complex than you thought, you're likely escaping life and hiding out in the *addiction zone*.

Endurance exercise should be a *tool* for solving problems, not the supposed solution to those problems.

Periodically Review Your Motives and Your Methods

On a quarterly basis, retake the self-tests in this book. If your priorities have changed significantly since last time, or even if there's a shift in your reasons for engaging in an endurance sport, it may be time to rethink your goals and perhaps consciously cut back a bit while you look for other real-life solutions to pressing problems.

Do not feel that by occassionally cutting back on your endurance activity you'll lose interest in it or you'll be undermining your resolves. Everyone needs vacations and holidays. A change once in a while can be refreshing and can be a catalyst for self-improvement. Don't be afraid to cut back on your training periodically, staying at a level that will maintain fitness but that will also give you some psychological rest from the stress of ambitious endurance training.

Your endurance activity isn't going anywhere, but without periodic rests from the stress of training, you won't be going anywhere either.

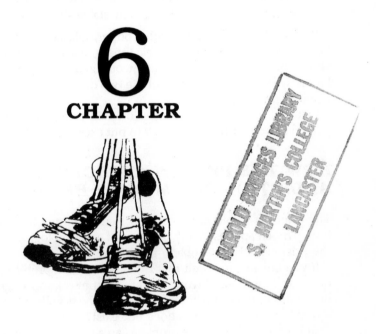

6
CHAPTER

HOW TO RECOVER FROM AEROBIC EXERCISE ADDICTION

What can be done to help a person deeply addicted to endurance sports? The treatment can take one of two directions:

1. Cure the affected person of all urge to participate in an endurance sport or activity, or

2. Modify the affected person's attitude and outlook so that he or she can continue to enjoy the benefits of endurance sports and activities, but at a level that is consistent with Glasser's positive addiction theories: in other words, at a level where the activities are firmly anchored on the psychologically stable side of the addiction lagoon.

Because I believe—along with Cooper, Glasser, and an army of other health professionals—that aerobic fitness, with its many proven benefits, should be not only tolerated but encouraged among the American population, we will ignore the first of the two directions: removing the person from all physical activity.

Instead, this chapter's discussion will center on what the addicted person can do for him- or herself to put exercising back on the right path.

HOW THE PERSON AFFECTED BY ADDICTION CAN MODIFY BEHAVIOR

The axiom is so old and overused that it sounds trite and hollow, but it very much applies to any problem of a psychological nature: To admit the existence of the problem is half the battle.

If you are able to admit that there is indeed a problem, half the battle has been fought—and won. Until the victim acknowledges the problem, no solution can be anticipated, because who is willing to work on solving a problem that—to them—does not exist?

Acknowledgment of the problem can also be a significant turning point because recognition, with exercise addiction, frequently involves some startling and severe insights about the self: insights that are sometimes painful and often starkly revealing, and that almost always spill over into a labyrinth of other psychological channels that have little to do with physical activity. Along with the revelation that you have a problem with your endurance pursuits often comes the realization that your overinvolvement in the sport is merely an outward sign of a tangle of confused reactions to the stresses, strains, and expectations of life.

If you truly feel that you have no problem, that your physical endurance endeavors are normal and healthy when in fact they are excessive and are having marked negative effects upon other aspects of your life, you won't have a start toward getting back on a reasonable, stable track. If you're lucky, a close friend or relative is more concerned about your welfare than you are and will stick by you and keep trying to work with you until you are ready for that all-important first step.

The first step is often taken unexpectedly.

The person deeply involved in exercise addiction often realizes a problem lurks at points in his or her training or racing or injury recovery. The realization sometimes comes as the blinding light came to Saul in the Bible.

A runner may be in the 19th mile of his 14th marathon of the year, fighting against gravity to stay upright and against inertia to keep moving, when the clouds part and there is a stark light surrounding a neon billboard that reads: *What Are You Doing To Yourself?*

Or a triathlete may come rushing into the bike-to-run transition area during her 10th triathlon in as many weeks, her bicycle cleats already hanging loosely from her pedals as she prepares to dismount in her socks to speed the transition. She sits down and dons her running shoes, rolls to her hands and knees, and pushes herself up during that awkward moment when the body attempts to make its own muscular transition from cycling to running on legs that are exhausted. Three steps later she stops dead in her tracks with a confused look on her face. The realization comes suddenly and profoundly: *I'm not really enjoying this. Why am I doing another one of these things so soon after the last one?*

In one way or another the revelation that something is wrong, something is out of gear, must come from within: the poignant moment when all rationalizations fall away and the glaring truth is apparent.

Frequently, this moment of illumination comes in the midst of a hard workout or a competition. Unfortunately, the affected person sometimes decides—out of learned habit—to continue with the workout or the race; the veil again descends, and the experience is written off to a lack of potassium or the heat or a momentary lapse in the steel-hard will to go on.

Remember Joe Oakes, whose realization came after he competed in the Ironman Triathlon with injuries from a recent car accident? He stopped for a while, trying to glue together the pieces, and made a major change in his attitude as a result.

"My attitude now is to try to enjoy it more," he said, "and not feel obligated to do things. I'm very selective about what I do. I won't do Ironman anymore, even though I love it. There are a thousand people there now, and it isn't the same for me.

"But the training is what is important now—the enjoyment of the training. I don't train for specific events. I may change my training once in a while. I like to keep myself at a high level of health. Not super race-ready. I can go out and do a race. I stay in shape that I could run a marathon, or a double marathon, whatever happens to come by. Or a quarter-mile run. I *love* quarter-mile runs. I did one this past weekend. I did it in 69 seconds, and you know, that's a square course; and if anyone had been near me, I'd have done 64 or 65."

Until the realization surfaces that a problem exists, however, you can do little for yourself. The work begins once the clouds part and the true reasons why you run, do triathlons, swim farther and faster are understood.

The challenge then is to overcome and peel away rationalizations that may have built up over time, while also modifying habits of training that you have worked to foster. Just as it is difficult to start an exercise program if you've never done one before, it is likewise difficult to slow down exercising when your motivation has been to increase so much and so quickly that you've become addicted along the way.

To modify an endurance-type exercise program takes at least as much intellectual and emotional stamina as it took to build your training to such an involved level in the first place. Fortunately, learning to do a 30-mile workout or a 1-hour swim in cold water developed certain talents for perseverance that you can also use to get off the exercise addiction merry-go-round. It takes the same talents—physical, emotional, psychological, and spiritual—to deliberately decrease workouts that it took to increase them, and if you're a victim of exercise addiction, you obviously have considerable talents upon which to draw.

Try a Radical Approach

The most extreme approach to gaining control of exercise addiction is like the cigarette smoker's technique of going cold turkey.

Simply stop.

As soon as you recognize your problem, go cold turkey and overnight turn into the epitome of the couch potato, the ultimate bump on the log.

For some people, this is the best and most workable solution.

Set up a specific time during which will just plain *stop!* to give your body and mind a holiday. Perhaps, since you don't want to get incredibly out of shape, the period could be 2 weeks. Two weeks is considered by most to be the point at which the fitness edge begins to melt. For some, however, it might better serve the purpose to take a month off. A month to do all of those things around the house that you've put off for so long; a month in which you read the Sunday paper from front to back; a month when you actually go to the movies instead of renting a tape of a recent film to which you can conveniently fall asleep while resting your eyes in your favorite easy chair.

Then, very carefully, you can *restart* your fitness program. This time, however, you'll start it up with some very firm guidelines in place before your first workout. Guidelines such as a limit on the time each day you'll devote to working out. Guidelines spelled out in a 3-month or 6-month or year-long program you've mapped out during an entirely rational period—a program that includes rest days and allows for a little modest racing if you want, but a program that is rational, logical, and humane instead of compulsive and driven.

The beauty of going cold turkey and then restarting is that with a month off, some of the battle wounds scar over, the mind has a chance to rest, and a certain stability descends. Then, when you *do* restart, the process, resumed at a starter's pace, can be a sort of rebirth, recalling the high points of beginning the first time around: the first 2-mile run, the first

Fun-Run, the first ultrashort triathlon followed by a celebration picnic with the family.

If you've been deeply addicted, going cold turkey may turn you off to exercising for several months. When you spend a few weeks away from the grind of exercising, you may find yourself remembering rather vividly some of the things you subjected yourself to and become repulsed by the activity; you may literally turn on it and, at least for a time, want no part of it. (This is a common reaction among compulsive people, obsessed with being into everything that's "in," who jumped on the running band-wagon and just *had* to run a marathon so that they could brag about it at cocktail parties, and who trained for 4 months, ran the marathon—usually quite badly—and never ran a step again.)

Create a Reasonable Level and Then Drop Back 15 Yards

If going cold turkey is not the best method for you—and for many it's not—you can simply sit down at the kitchen table with a tablet and begin laying out a reasonable training program to which you can fall back. This program should build in hard/easy/easy days, rest days, cross training, and enough flexibility that if you miss a scheduled day, no sweaty palms and no urges to make it up ensue. The schedule *can* include several race dates—especially if those dates are heavy with sentimental value: a race you've run every year since its inception, a race that falls on your favorite holiday or near your birthday—but your race schedule and your training schedule should be cut at least in half!

This modified schedule allows for a reasonable level to which you can revert as a base. You can stay fit, your injuries can begin healing, and you can become a social animal again instead of a workout animal. You may wish to stay at that level for several months as you rethink your ratio-nale for exercising, your motivations, and your long-term plans. Then, when you decide to increase your exercise program, do so at a very reason-able rate: 5 percent per year.

This seems, at first glance, outrageously modest. But it isn't. It is a rate that many of the world's best coaches advise for their world-class ath-letes. And it is a rate they certainly advise for amateurs.*

---

*With 10 or 15 years of base behind them, world-class athletes who've worked on long-term programs may be doing 90 miles of running a week, and a 5 percent increase might put them up to 94.5 miles. This seems incredibly high to the novice, but it is relatively se-date against the background the athlete has built over many, many years. By contrast, an amateur athlete jumping from 20 miles a week to 30 is, according to the world's best coaches, asking for trouble because of the high percentage of the jump in mileage—an incredible 50 percent. Once again, it comes back to battling the typical American's unwillingness to be patient and the desire for quick results: that is, instant gratification.

Doug Latimer, Mr. Western States, reflected on a change in attitude induced by a reformulated program: "I've changed my attitude a lot. I've become much more casual, but it [Western States] is still my main goal. I would love to have the time to train aggressively to really try to win the race, or to be second or third again, which I have not been able to do the last 2 or 3 years. But I would not be nearly as compulsive. I've learned, for example, that not only is it okay to take a day off in the middle of serious training, it's very beneficial to take some time off. If you run 40 or 50 miles of Western States–type training one day and you're beat, to do your obligatory 6 or 7 miles the next day, even if it's at an easy pace, just isn't always good. Your body recovers much better if you don't run at all the day after a hard run than if you go out and do a light jog.

"I used to run 3 or 4 months in training for Western States at 125 miles a week on the average, and never miss a day. Last year [1986] I went to the other extreme and probably underdid it. My training consisted of a longish run on the weekend and maybe two midweek runs, one of which would be somewhat a hilly run, but a short run, and the other would be just a jog. So I was running three, at most four times a week and my top week was 83 miles. That was not enough but it was adequate, and you don't need to be nearly as compulsive about training as hard as most people do. If I knew then what I know now, I would probably have won the race 4 years in a row. Because of combinations of stupid training, stupid pacing, and stupid nutrition, it cost me at least two races.

"I think that right now, I have a pretty good perspective. I want to keep running because I love it and because it is good for you. It is an important part of my life's plan. If I give up running, number one, I feel I would die a lot sooner, and number two, I think I would not be as healthy as I approach the end as I will be if I keep running. So I value it for that reason, but I am really not compulsive. I still have goals. I would like to be running a lot more than I am, but the fact that I am not is because I have put it in perspective. Now if I have to get that letter out, or that memo out, I do that and the running comes second. Or, if I haven't seen my kids for a while or my wife enough, then instead of going out for that run that will get me home late for dinner, I'll skip it and get home on time for the family dinner. So I think that, yes, it is finally in perspective."

When you draw up your new program, make it a long-term one. If you can work out your program for a full year, that's excellent. Then, after 6 months, if you can draw up the 6 months out beyond the first year, terrific! This method keeps *you* in control of your program. It puts *you* in the driver's seat instead of making you the slave to whatever compulsion happens to strike you, and damn the program.

Seek Out Persons Who've Come Through Similar Experiences

Because psychologically based problems are so personal and so all-consuming, the affected person tends to feel unique in the world. Or, even more disheartening, to feel that he or she is the only one who has *ever* experienced this problem.

Nothing could be farther from the truth.

Although each of us is, in our own way, unique, we are not unique to the point where we have nothing in common with other people. On the contrary: When it comes to problems, many, many people find that they have very much in common with others.

A person experiencing exercise addiction is not the first person to have such an experience. Consider Joe Oakes or Doug Latimer. Also consider that for this discussion, they were drawn from a very limited geographic area. Oakes lives 12 miles from Latimer. I did not have to scour the countryside to find examples.

Within a reasonable distance there is bound to be someone else who has gone through many of the problems associated with exercise addiction that you are going through. Getting in contact with such a person would be valuable.

Not that the other person can provide a cure, but he or she will almost certainly be able to offer observations on coming back to the center after spending months or years over the edge. Moreover, people who have shared your problems can reassure you that what you are experiencing is not unique, it is not overwhelming, it is not something that can't be coped with or beaten. These people have the unique distinction of having been there and come back safely. Nothing you can say will surprise them. And besides, they'll probably be able to tell you stories that will further assure you that your situation is not hopeless.

The act of seeking help from others who have had similar experience works wonders at Alcoholics Anonymous (AA), and it can have similar good effects in the case of exercise addiction. It is also very consoling to know that, once a contact is established, there is someone a phone call away who will at least understand your plight.

Where do you find such people?

Generally, they are well known within their athletic circles because their outrageous exploits have given them a sort of notoriety. If you are a runner, contact the president or secretary of a local running club. Cyclists can contact officers of local cycling clubs and organizations. The same goes for swimmers, triathletes, and other endurance athletes. Every club officer knows of one or more—sometimes many—athletes who went overboard and invariably made their way back to a healthier, happier center.

Ask for the names and phone numbers of people who went overboard but managed to return to their sport with a *healthy* outlook. Avoid talking to people who went overboard and subsequently dropped out of their sport. These people are frequently embittered by the experience and are usually the wrong people to ask for a sympathetic ear or a helping hand.

Diversify Your Aerobic Sports Approach or Substitute

If you are determined to kick the habit yourself instead of asking for outside assistance, one method that can help break up the habit is to ease other aerobic sports into your regimen.

If you are a runner, throw in some cycling or some rope jumping or low-impact aerobic dance. This method is not easy; addicted athletes seem to have a built-in resistance to changing sports. It is almost as though they feel that they are being unfaithful to the sport they've grown to love.

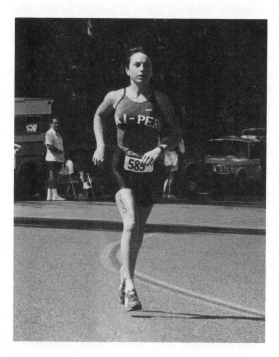

Rhonda Provost, a Northern California triathlete, admits to having become obsessive during the first several years of her triple-training. A veteran of the "Escape from Alcatraz" and 6 half-Ironman distance triathlons, she now competes in 2 to 3 triathlons a year, with (at least) the season-ending "Bass Lake Classic Triathlon" done purely for fun. (Richard Benyo photograph)

But the process of changing sports is not unlike the process of getting involved in the original sport in the first place. The new sport has to be eased into gradually; it must be carefully fitted into one's schedule and practiced on a regular basis.

There is a danger in this, of course. Using other aerobic or endurance sports to break the habit of the sport that has become your obsession may simply create additional obsessions. You may end up becoming a triathlete or a quadrathlete or worse. Frequently, however, by breaking up the obsessive outlook toward the singular sport, you can break loose of it and manage to reintegrate it into your life on a new, controlled basis.

If diversifying to several different endurance sports does not work, you might try to substitute a different aerobic sport (particularly one you feel you are not especially fond of) to take the place of the one that has gotten out of hand.

The very act of learning a new sport while easing out of the obsessing sport frequently brings the original activity down in volume and intensity to a point where you can remember the fun it used to be when you practiced it at a much more reasonable level.

Moreover, by taking up a different endurance sport, you can begin to remedy some of the physical problems (such as injuries) that are usually associated with the too frequent practice of one sport. This way of alleviating some of the discomfort caused by the obsessing sport will help wean you away from the original stressor.

Unfortunately, there is a risk of the addiction merely being transferred from one sport to another. But this need not be the case. Developing the new sport provides an opportunity to set up guidelines for heading off addiction and offers a new beginning, from which you can do it right.

Allow the Social Animal Within You to Have Its Head

The human is a social animal, despite the way some of us rationalize our need to be alone. Even the person with a genuine need for considerable solitude occasionally needs to be around and communicate with people. And a shy person may be shy not because he or she wishes to be, but because he or she has failed—for whatever reason—to develop the mechanisms necessary for comfortable socializing with others.

Although endurance sports offer some camaraderie, and although that camaraderie can include some of the most profound relationships in a person's life, the essence of endurance sports is going it alone. Endurance sports are unlike team sports, in which you must train with others to develop cooperative skills. They are unlike one-on-one games or sports such as bowling, chess, tennis, or racquetball. The distance runner, triathlete, or endurance swimmer competes mainly against him- or herself. Sure, there may be a field of 10,000 in a marathon, but you typically compete against your personal record (PR) and therefore against yourself. In an endurance swim, no other competitor may be present: It may be you against the English Channel or you against the cold and the currents between Alcatraz Island and the shoreline at Aquatic Park in San Francisco.

As part of your program of re-entry into the real world and out of the "spaced-out state" of exercise addiction, reestablish friendships, first at home with family and friends, then with coworkers and old acquaintances. And do so with an eye—and an ear—toward what *their* interests are. In many cases, your family and friends have supported you during your obsessive competitions, often doubling as support crews and spectators for your endurance endeavors, even when doing so interfered with their plans. Take time to pay them back for their dedication by showing some interest in their activities and concerns.

Maybe you've missed most of your kids' baseball and soccer games because you had to train. Make it a point to attend as many games as you can; support their efforts. Pitch in a bit around the house, not as a martyr, but as a participant interested in what goes on around you.

Get together with friends to watch them play softball and go for a beer afterward. Or go with a friend to an art gallery opening, even if you think you won't enjoy it. You've been so immersed in training for so long that little else has entered your consciousness. Now that you're trying to get onto an even keel, attempt to flood your consciousness with other things that are happening with your family and friends and in your community. Besides serving to resocialize you, they'll keep you occupied and your mind off training.

If one reason you originally got involved in endurance sports was that you are a solitary person, make an effort to mingle with people, even if it means going solo to a movie or a concert. Or take the time you would have spent in obsessive training to read a book you've been curious about or to take up playing an instrument. Redirect some of your energies. Just do *something* to fill the space you would have devoted to training, so that you don't sit around dwelling on its loss.

Reestablish Old Interests to Occupy Training Time

For some people who have become too involved in endurance sports, the time spent running or swimming or cycling or cross-country skiing filled a very real vacuum in life. For others, the time needed to get overinvolved in an aerobic sport replaced a negative addiction. And for still others, the time needed to become addicted to a sport and to then take it out of bounds replaced time that was previously spent doing something else, whether it was stamp collecting or ballroom dancing, watching TV game shows or bowling.

Because endurance sports taken to the extreme do consume such a tremendous amount of time, they almost always force *something* else out of the exerciser's life.

If that something was not an activity that was detrimental to you, reestablishing an interest in that activity, at first gently and then with more fervor, is a viable way to fill the time once spent in training and to ease the possible symptoms of withdrawal from the aerobic activity. A person who is genuinely busy has less time to dwell on the pains and pangs of withdrawal.

This method of easing out of an aerobic addiction can—and should— interact with other solutions.

Often, the activity that was deserted involved other people. Reestablishing contact with the abandoned activity and the people associated with it can greatly lessen the pain of easing out of an unhealthy aerobic lifestyle. The interaction with other people, the socializing (as with the previous method), can greatly soften the trauma of withdrawing from the all-consuming endurance sport.

Develop Other Interests to Take Your Mind Off Training

If, indeed, your aerobic activity filled a vacuum in your life, you can compensate for its loss by developing other, new interests.

Everyone has *something* they've always wanted to do. What would you do well if you were to apply to it the kind of energy you poured into your aerobic obsession?

It's never too late to learn to play a musical instrument, study a foreign language, take up carpentry or gardening, get involved in volunteer work or political groups—or even offer to coach young people in your aerobic sport, if you feel you must maintain some involvement with it.

Be Firm With Yourself in Establishing Goals

This counsel harkens back to the previous chapter on how to avoid exercise addiction in the first place. Even if you are deeply involved in exercise addiction, you can put the brakes on a runaway program by setting goals, especially short-term goals.

The very act of formulating goals on blank paper places boundaries around your program, which tends to bring it back under your power.

The process also may be intimidating in that you are likely to take a hard look at your current program in the context of a system of goals.

The very act of asking yourself, "Just what are my goals, anyway?" frequently serves as a jolt, because the athlete who is addicted often has only vague, fuzzy goals or none at all.

The absence of goals indicates the absence of a coherent program. The realization that you lack a coherent program may make you question your motives for exercising and can point up rationalizations upon which the exercising was built.

But even if the setting of short-term goals has no such dramatic effect, it can still force some logic and common sense into an often pointless exercise program.

In taking the time to consult some of the better training books available and in formulating viable short-term goals, you will realize that your existing "program" does not seem to mesh with anything advised by those who are accomplished and credible in the sport.

"Addictive people, I think, lose the perception of what it is they're doing," stated marathoner Nancy Ditz. "And that's why I think that if they sit down, today, and plan out what it is they're going to do, it'll make a difference. There are hundreds of books and magazines that you can consult about running or exercise. And if you consult them and lay out a program, it's a framework in which you'll be obliged to work.

"And then there's also the admonition to 'listen to your body,' which everyone talks about but which few people do well. You've got to measure out all the things in your life: your work, your family, your other recreational activities, how much sleep you get, how much time you spend commuting. And they're all factors in your *complete* life, and they all impact on your training—and they *should* impact your training, because your training is *part* of your life, not your whole life."*

Be Patient, For Your Body Will Eventually Break Down

If one pattern emerges in previous chapters of this book, it is that eventually something happens to some people that knocks them out of the brush with exercise addiction. The precipitating stress causes some of these people to modify their behavior; in more radical cases, an injury

---

*The potential problem with a precise, well-researched, proven program is that a perfectly intelligent person can adopt such a program and, while ignoring several critical aspects of the program—usually involving scheduled rest days, and so on—can assume that it is being followed to the letter and is just not working for him or her. Or the user may conclude that the author of the program, perhaps an Olympic champion, just does not understand the person's body as well as he or she does.

causes them to stop their physical activity entirely for a time before getting back onto the right track.

Since most people who become addicted to exercise are not elite or world-class athletes, a built-in safety valve is involved. That safety valve is the fact that exercise addiction victims are seldom endowed with genes or biomechanics that raise them to world-class level or protect them from physical problems and difficulties.

Consequently, since these people take on so much physical activity so quickly and continue to escalate that activity beyond all common sense, their chances of encountering serious physical difficulties—in the way of injuries and exhaustion—are extremely high. In this respect, a built-in braking device ultimately prevents them from going any farther, thereby disconnecting their addiction.

Certainly, many amateur endurance athletes continue to train through injuries and other adversities. They continually damage themselves until they reach the point where they are no longer able to participate in their sport.

In most cases, however, once the ability to pursue the physical activity is removed, the person goes through a period of depression and then a period of anger. Ironically, the anger is not directed inward. Instead, it is often directed at the sport pursued so irrationally, as though the sport were responsibile for what happened, and not the user. The person perceives him- or herself as a victim of the unfeeling cruelty of the sport.

So, if nothing suggested previously in this chapter seems to work to free you from the bonds of exercise addiction, just keep up your current pace and your body will step in to bring your career to a conclusion.

This theory of being patient and waiting for the cycle to complete itself is one that world-class runner Rod Dixon of New Zealand believes in. Dixon is one of the few men in the world to have run both sub-4-minute miles and a sub-2:10 marathon. I had the opportunity to speak with Dixon and asked him how he would handle an exercise-addicted person.

"Those people are quite easy—especially if they've gone up and over. You get them on the way up where they are seeing this incredible improvement. Initially, when they started, they couldn't run around the block, but now they can run around the block 10 times without sweating. Now they're running from one town to the other and their 10K time has come down. They're very difficult to work with, they've gone overboard. But it comes around in cycles. Eventually they come back by themselves."

Latimer expressed a similar view: "I think people have to find out for themselves. It's like telling someone in the first stages of infatuation with a new girlfriend or boyfriend, telling them that this may not be the girl of their dreams because she isn't educated or she has bad teeth, or whatever it might be. They are not going to see it. They have to burn themselves through. But I would say something [to them] and counsel them to be moderate and take the long view. But they wouldn't pay any attention.''

Unfortunately, waiting until you break down to the point that you can no longer train or compete is a radical solution. In most instances, however, it is the ultimate solution—a solution provided by the body itself, almost in self-defense. Certainly, it is possible to explore another avenue before things reach the point where they take care of themselves by immobilizing you.

Seek Professional Help

A decade ago, I'm not so sure I'd have been willing to suggest seeking professional psychological help for a problem like exercise addiction, primarily because so few psychologists and psychiatrists were aware of the psychology behind endurance sports. In the mid-1970s, for example, there were probably fewer than a dozen professionals in this country who appreciated the unique psychological problems encountered by the amateur endurance athlete. Even those dozen or so professionals who were genuinely interested in the subject were still poking and probing about, trying to find answers to baffling questions concerning what happened to the mind when a person ran 90 miles a week.

Today, however, I feel confident in suggesting to people who suspect they are suffering from exercise addiction that they seek the help of a professional specializing in sports psychology. Most major metropolitan centers have a good supply of such specialists: psychologists and psychiatrists who run, cycle, do triathlons, or do endurance swimming themselves, and who are very much interested in the subject. They are concerned about helping athletes overcome performance blocks, helping amateur athletes build confidence in their own abilities, helping them reconcile their professional lives with the things they learn about themselves from participating in endurance sports. And most of those practitioners are qualified to help someone who overindulges in an endurance sport to first throttle back a bit, and to then explore the psychological dynamics that caused the compulsion to go overboard in the first place.

The problem most often has little, if anything, to do with the endurance sport itself; the sport is merely the vehicle that the person uses to express the compulsion. Unfortunately, the endurance sport, being essentially positive, can be difficult to shake because its use—unlike negative addictions such as drugs or gambling—can easily be justified in terms of its many health and fitness benefits.

If you feel your tendency toward compulsion is surfacing in your training and racing, it is good advice to seek psychological help well before the compulsion escalates to the level of abject addiction. If it has already escalated, and if you are able to take the step of acknowledging the problem, consult a competent professional specializing in sport.

Your family doctor may be able to suggest an appropriate specialist. If not, contact the *American College of Sports Medicine, P.O. Box 1440, Indianapolis, IN 46206,* for a listing of their members in your area. You may have to travel to a nearby city in order to meet with one of these specialists, but we're talking about your psychological well-being, which affects your physical well-being, and it is worth it—before your body breaks down badly enough to pull the plug on you.

EPILOGUE: ON THE ROAD AGAIN

To some, it might seem radical to advise a person who has become healthy through aerobic exercise to consult a psychologist or psychiatrist. In discussing the subject of this book with fellow amateur athletes over more than a decade, I frequently found it amusing that some of the most hardcore and addicted athletes felt comfortable in commenting, "So-and-So is going overboard, don't you think? He really ought to see somebody about this. What he's doing with his running is only a symptom of something that runs much deeper, you know?"

They were correct, of course. The person in question had, more often than not, come to running from some other activity that allowed a similar pattern of obsessive-compulsive behavior to billow up. The human, in that regard, is so diverse and creative as to stagger the imagination. One runner I met and joined for some long Saturday workouts in the late 1970s was in the process of becoming compulsive about running while shedding a compulsiveness about disco dancing. During the crossover period, when he went disco dancing from Friday night at 8 until 3 in the morning and then got up at 7 to meet me for an 18-mile workout, he was one pooped-out cowboy. Although I have no psychological training, I don't think I was far off the mark in figuring that the poor fellow was desperately looking for himself, searching for an image that he liked and found socially uplifting, into which he could pour a personality that he wasn't especially comfortable with as he'd nurtured it.

Certainly, not everyone who goes overboard in some activity—and who, in fact, becomes compulsive in that activity—needs psychological help. Some people are in the process of growing, of exploring alternatives in life, of looking for something within themselves with which they'll be comfortable. Some just happen to have compulsive personalities that dictate that whatever they do, they do it full speed ahead.

For too many of the people I have run with, the end to the running addiction was a simple one: injury.

This was usually due to the fact that they'd taken up running later in life, and their bodies had had no breaking in period; they just plain overused certain body parts until they ran them into the ground, broken. Or their bodies were not biomechanically correct for running—they'd have been better off in professional wrestling—and once again, something gave out. Injury was most often the route to breaking the addiction.

As I've indicated elsewhere in this book, too frequently the debilitating injuries have turned a gung-ho athletic enthusiast into one of the sport's staunchest critics—not unlike the former smoker whose passionate stand against smoking far outstrips that of the antismoker who has never tasted nicotine.

Fortunately, most of the people I knew who left the sport through injury and had to be numbered among the sport's harshest critics eventually worked their way back into a lifestyle of aerobic fitness. But they came back in a much more tentative way, as though, on the second go-round, being careful to take from the sport the best it had to offer: Once burned, they were extremely careful to keep the right foot from ever again flooring the accelerator.

Although my own obsessiveness with long-distance running produced its share of injuries, none was ever quite serious enough to make me stop entirely. The closest I came to a chronic injury was a series of upper Achilles tendon problems that cropped up like clockwork near Thanksgiving each year and that I had to nurse into January by taking days off and by alternating running workouts with bicycle riding. Perhaps I was spared the one big serious injury because I'd run a lot as a kid and because I'd run cross-country in college and was relatively sound biomechanically.

My own chance to get off the aerobic rollercoaster came about by the accident that I've already mentioned, wherein I decided to substitute quality for quantity. After running eight marathons in as many months in 1978 and never breaking 3:22, I decided to alter my training by building toward a specific race. I ran a 3:11 in early 1979, then a 3:05 later in the year. Heartened by the results of some of the changes I'd adopted, I radically altered my training in 1980, weaning myself from long, long runs every weekend and going to the track for speed workouts twice a week. I ran only three marathons in 1980, two of them (a 3:30 in June and a 3:19 in July) as a concession to friends who planned to run them, but also as a concession to myself: I used them as calculated long workouts. In early October I ran a 2:57 that went so well throughout that I ran overly conservatively, believing that at some point it had to unravel; it never did.

The hard training for my first sub-3:00 race taught me that running is a tool and an outlet, not a separate entity that has power to make me do things that, under more sober circumstances, I would never contemplate.

Since then I've managed to relegate running to the status of an important ingredient in my life, but not *the* overwhelming ingredient. I still run a marathon or two a year, always under 3:30 and sometimes near 3:00; but because my running now is more relaxed and less obsessive, the sub-3:30s come on less mileage than they did a decade ago, and those near 3:00 come without the single-minded intensity I had in 1980.

There are still occasionally runs that border on the sublime, on the mystical, but they are run without a half hour of warming up to mask semi-injured tendons. And the lack of obsession with running has opened some time for more serious bicycling, which I must admit that my body enjoys as it grows older: My body finds nothing unpalatable in a workout on a bicycle where my feet never touch the road, and the road in turn never gets a chance to pound my feet, ankles, legs, and tendons.

But perhaps most important, the perspective that I've now got on my running—one in which obsessiveness is not necessary to make things work—has washed over into other aspects of life. Quality, indeed, is better than quantity. And often, less is more.

REFERENCES

Bird, P. (1987, September). Runner's high revisited. *Triathlete,* pp. 18, 66-67.

Brant, J. (1986, April). Beyond ultra. *Outside,* pp. 70-72, 110-112.

Cantrell, G. (1985, November). How slow is too slow? *Ultrarunning,* p. 14.

Carmack, M., & Martens, R. (1979). Measuring commitment to running: A survey of runners' attitudes and mental states. *Journal of Sports Psychology,* **1**, 25-42.

Chan, C. (1986). Addicted to exercise. *Encyclopedia Brittanica Medical and Health Annual* (pp. 429-432).

Chan, C., & Grossman, H. (1988). Psychological effects of running loss on consistent runners. *Perceptual and Motor Skills,* **66**, 875-883.

Cooper, K. (1968). *Aerobics.* New York: Evans.

Gallup, A. (Ed.) (1987). *Gallup leisure activities index.* Princeton, NJ: The Gallup Polls.

Glasser, W. (1976). *Positive addiction.* New York: Harper & Row.

Higdon, H. (1978, January). Can running cure mental illness? Part 1. *Runner's World,* pp. 36-43.

Higdon, H. (1978, February). Can running cure mental illness? Part 2. *Runner's World,* pp. 36-43.

Hughes, J. & Kosterlitz, H. (1975). *Nature* magazine. London, England.

Johnson, H. (reporter). (July 12, 1988). *Running and Racing* [videotape]. Atlanta, GA: ESPN.

Kasch, F., Wallace, J., Van Camp, S., & Verity, L. (1988). A longitudinal study of cardiovascular stability in active men aged 45 to 65 years. *The Physician and Sportsmedicine,* **16**(1), 117-126.

Kavanagh, T. (1986). *The healthy heart program.* Emmaus, PA: Rodale Press.

Kostrubala, T. (1976). *The joy of running.* Philadelphia: Lippincott.

Layman, D. (1986). *The runner: A profile of injury and addiction.* Urbana, IL: University of Illinois.

Lunder, R. (1988, May 3). Once is never enough for prisoners of compulsion. *San Jose Mercury News.* pp. E1, E2.

McCunney, R. (1987). Fitness, heart disease, and high-density lipoproteins: A look at the relationships. *The Physician and Sportsmedicine,* **15**(2), 67-79.

McNair, P.M., Lorr, M., & Droppleman. (1971). *Profile of mood states.* San Diego, CA: Educational & Industrial Testing Service.

Morgan, D., Cruise, R., Girardin, B., Lutz-Schneider, V., Morgan, D., & Qi, W. (1986). HDL-C concentrations in weight-trained, endurance-trained, and sedentary females. *The Physician and Sportsmedicine,* **14**(3), 166-181.

Myturn. (July 11, 1988). *Newsweek.* p. 52.

Nieman, D. (1986). *The sports medicine fitness course.* Palo Alto, CA: Bull Publishing.

Oldridge, N.B. (1982). Compliance and exercise in primary and secondary prevention of coronary heart disease: A review. *Preventive Medicine,* **11**(1), 56-70.

Paffenbarger, R., Hyde, R., Wing, A., & Hsieh, C-C. (1986). Physical activity, all-case mortality, and longevity of college alumni. *New England Journal of Medicine,* **314**, 605-613.

Rippe, J. (Ed.) (1987a). The health benefits of exercise: Part 1. *The Physician and Sportsmedicine,* **15**(10), 114-132.

Rippe, J. (Ed.) (1987b). The health benefits of exercise: Part 2. *The Physician and Sportsmedicine,* **15**(11), 120-131.

Rosenberg, M. (1965). *Society and the adolescent self-image.* Princeton, NJ: Princeton University.

Zailian, M. (1986, May 4). On the edge: Dern breaks a Dipsea barrier. *San Francisco Chronicle.* p. 31.

Zung, W. (1965). A self-rating depression scale. *Archives of General Psychiatry,* **12**, 63-70.

SUGGESTED
READINGS

Benjamin, B. (1984). *Listen to your pain.* New York: Penguin.

Cooper, K. (1985). *Running without fear.* New York: Bantam.

Corbin, C., & Lindsey, R. (1984). *The ultimate fitness book.* Champaign, IL: Leisure Press.

Costill, D. (1979). *A scientific approach to distance running.* Los Altos, CA: Tafnews.

Csikszentmihalyi, M. (1988). *Beyond boredom and anxiety.* San Francisco: Jossey-Bass.

Daly, D. (1987, August 3). An endurance of marathon quality. *Insight,* pp. 50-52.

Duda, M. (1987). High endorphin levels mask silent ischemia? *The Physician and Sportsmedicine,* **15**(3), 40.

Eichner, E. (1986). Coagulability and rheology: Hematologic benefits from exercise, fish, and aspirin. Implications for athletes and nonathletes. *The Physician and Sportsmedicine,* **14**(10), 102-110.

Elman, J. (1986, July). The loneliest of the long-distance runners. *Runner's World,* pp. 34-39.

Elrick, H., Crakes, J., & Clarke, S. (1978). *Living longer & better: Guide to optimal health.* Mountain View, CA: World Publications.

Friedman, R. (1986). Nature's link between pleasure and pain. *Stanford Medicine,* **3**(3), 28-32.

Hanson, P. (1986). *The joy of stress.* Kansas City: Andrews, McMeel & Parker.

Haskell, W., Camargo, C., Williams, P., Vranizan, K., Krauss, R., Lingren, F., & Wood, P. (1984). The effect of cessation and resumption of moderate alcohol intake on serum high-density-lipoprotein subfractions. *New England Journal of Medicine,* **310**, 805-810.

Higdon, H. (1984, November). Jim Fixx: How he lived, why he died. *The Runner,* pp. 32-38.

Kalyn, W. (1985, October). Aerobics with a kick. *Esquire,* pp. 51-52.

Lane, N., Bloch, D., Jones, H., Marshall, W., Wood, P., & Fries, J. (1986). Long-distance running, bone density and osteoarthritis. *Journal of the American Medical Association,* **255**, 1147-1151.

Lane, N., Bloch, D., Wood, P., & Fries, J. (1987). Aging, long-distance running, and the development of musculoskeletal disability. *American Journal of Medicine,* **82,** 772-780.

Leonard, G. (1987, May) Mastery: The secret of ultimate fitness. *Esquire,* pp. 113-116.

Miller, B., Galton, L., & Brunner, D. (1972). *Freedom from heart attacks.* New York: Simon & Schuster.

Monahan, T. (1986a). From activity to eternity. *The Physician and Sportsmedicine,* **14**(6), 156-164.

Monahan, T. (1986b). Should women go easy on exercise? *The Physician and Sportsmedicine,* **14**(12), 188-197.

Monahan, T. (1987). Treating athletic amenorrhea: A matter of instinct? *The Physician and Sportsmedicine,* **15**(7), 184-189.

Moore, R., & Webb, G. (1986). *The K factor.* New York: Macmillan.

Nash, H. (1987). Do compulsive runners and anorectic patients share common bonds? *The Physician and Sportsmedicine,* **15**(12), 162-167.

Paffenbarger, R., Brand, R., Sholtz, R., & Jung, D. (1978). Energy expenditure, cigarette smoking, and blood pressure level as related to death from specific diseases. *American Journal of Epidemiology,* **108,** 12-18.

Paffenbarger, R., Hale, W., Brand, R., & Hyde, R. (1977). Work-energy level, personal characteristics, and fatal heart attack: A birth-cohort effect. *American Journal of Epidemiology,* **105,** 200-213.

Paffenbarger, R., Wing, A., & Hyde, R. (1978). Physical activity as an index of heart attack risk in college alumni. *American Journal of Epidemiology,* **108,** 161-175.

Powell, K., Kohl, H., Caspersen, C., & Blair, S. (1986). An epidemiological perspective on the causes of running injuries. *The Physician and Sportsmedicine,* **14**(6), 100-114.

Rowan, R. (1986). *How to control high blood pressure without drugs.* New York: Scribners.

Sachs, M., & Buffone, G. (Eds.) (1984). *Running as therapy: An integrated approach.* Lincoln, NE: University of Nebraska Press.

Shangold, M. (1986). How I manage exercise-related menstrual disturbances. *The Physician and Sportsmedicine,* **14**(3), 113-120.

Sheehan, G. (1975). *Dr. Sheehan on running.* Mountain View, CA: World Publications.

Shulman, N., Saunders, E., & Hall, W. (1987). *High blood pressure.* New York: Macmillan.

Simon, H., & Levisohn, S. (1987). *The athlete within.* Boston: Little, Brown & Company.

Smith, E., & Gilligan, C. (1987). Effects of inactivity and exercise on bone. *The Physician and Sportsmedicine,* **15**(11), 91-102.

Steinman, D. (1983, October). Life in the fast lane—one step ahead of the devil. *Runner's World Quarterly*, pp. 48-54.

Tipton, C. (1987). Commentary: Physicians should advise wrestlers about weight loss. *The Physician and Sportsmedicine*, **15**(1), 160-165.

INDEX

ABOUT
THE AUTHOR

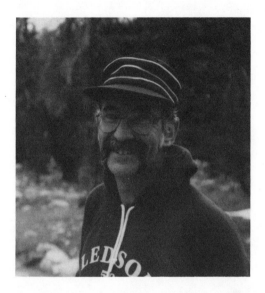

Richard Benyo is no stranger to the literary world or the world of aerobic exercise. As the former executive editor of *Runner's World* magazine, he has seen and experienced the gruesome side of exercise addiction. Only Richard Benyo could express the feelings of an exercise addict with such literary flair, having been a marathon junkie but truly overcoming the pain and entrapment of exercise addiction.

Benyo is now a fitness and running columnist for the *San Francisco Chronicle*. He is the author of numerous health and fitness books, including *Masters of the Marathon* and *Elaine LaLanne's Fitness After 50*, and the editor of *The Complete Woman Runner*. He has also written articles for *American Health*, *Popular Computing*, and *The New Yorker*.

Richard Benyo resides in the Napa Valley of Northern California, and enjoys running, reading, and collecting and listening to '50s and '60s rock 'n' roll music.